Nursing the Acutely Ill Adult

Case Book

Case Book Series

This book is part of a new series of case books written for nursing and other allied health profession students. The books are designed to help students link theory and practice and provide an engaging and focused way to learn.

Titles published in this series:

Paramedics: From Street to Emergency Department Case Book
Sarah Fellows and Bob Fellows

Midwifery: Emergencies, Critical Illness and Incidents Case Book
Maureen Raynor, Jayne Marshall and Karen Jackson

Mental Health Nursing Case Book
Edited by Nick Wrycraft

Learning Disability Case Book
Edited by Bob Hallawell

Nursing the Acutely Ill Adult Case Book
Karen Page and Aiden McKinney

Perioperative Practice Case Book
Paula Strong and Suzanne Hughes

Visit www.openup.co.uk/casebooks for information and sample chapters from other books in the series.

Nursing the Acutely Ill Adult

Case Book

**Edited by
Karen Page and
Aidín McKinney**

Open University Press

Open University Press
McGraw-Hill Education
McGraw-Hill House
Shoppenhangers Road
Maidenhead
Berkshire
England
SL6 2QL

email: enquiries@openup.co.uk
world wide web: www.openup.co.uk

and Two Penn Plaza, New York, NY 10121-2289, USA

First published 2012

A catalogue record of this book is available from the British Library

ISBN-13: 978-0-33-524309-9 (pb)
ISBN-10: 0-33-524309-6 (pb)
eISBN: 978-0-33-524310-5

Library of Congress Cataloging-in-Publication Data
CIP data applied for

Typesetting and e-book compilations by
RefineCatch Limited, Bungay, Suffolk
Printed and bound in the UK by Ashford Colour Press Ltd, Gosport, Hampshire

The McGraw·Hill Companies

Contents

List of figures

List of tables

Notes on contributors

Patrick Gallagher is currently employed as a Teaching Fellow based in the School of Nursing and Midwifery at Queens University Belfast. He is involved in the delivery of a variety of modules to undergraduate nursing students. He has extensive experience as a Registered Nurse specializing in cardiology and is the course director for the Immediate Life Support (ILS) course and coordinates delivery of the ILS course to all adult field nursing students. His main research interests include improving outcomes of critically ill patients through educational means.

Niall McKenna is currently employed as a Teaching Fellow based in the School of Nursing and Midwifery at Queens University Belfast. He is involved in the delivery of a variety of modules to undergraduate nursing students. He is an ILS instructor and delivers the Immediate Life Support (ILS) course. His teaching responsibilities include pathophysiology, pharmacology, the care of the acutely ill patient and a post-registration course specializing in cardiology.

Billie Joan Rice is currently employed as a Teaching Fellow based in the School of Nursing and Midwifery at Queens University Belfast. She is involved in the delivery of a variety of modules to undergraduate nursing students. She has extensive experience as a Registered Nurse specializing in cardiology. She is an ILS instructor and delivers the Immediate Life Support (ILS) course. Her teaching responsibilities include pathophysiology, pharmacology and the care of the acutely ill patient.

List of abbreviations

A&E Accident and Emergency
ABCDE Airway, Breathing, Circulation, Disability, Exposure
ABGs arterial blood gases
ACEI angiotensin-converting enzyme inhibitor
ACS acute coronary syndrome
ADH anti-diuretic hormone
ADP adenosine diphosphate
ADQI Acute Dialysis Quality Initiative
AEDs anti-epileptic drugs
AF atrial fibrillation
AHA American Heart Association
AKI acute kidney injury
AKIN Acute Kidney Injury Network
AML acute myeloid leukaemia
ANP atrial natriuretic peptide
APACHE acute physiology, age, chronic health evaluation
aPPT activated partial prothrombin time
ARDS adult respiratory distress syndrome
ARF acute renal failure
AST aspartate aminotransferase
ATN acute tubular necrosis
AVPU alert, can respond to voice, pain or is unresponsive
BMR basal metabolic rate
BNP brain natriuretic peptide
BP blood pressure
BSA body surface area
BUN blood urea nitrogen
cAMP cyclic adenosine monophosphate
CBF cerebral blood flow
CHD coronary heart disease
CHF chronic heart failure
CNP C-type natriuretic peptide
CNS central nervous system
COPD chronic obstructive pulmonary disease
CPP cerebral perfusion pressure
CPR cardiopulmonary resuscitation

CRP C-reactive protein
CRT capillary refill time
CSF cerebrospinal fluid
CT computed tomography
CTPA computed tomographic pulmonary angiograpy
CVP central verous pressure
CXR chest X-ray
DKA diabetic ketoacidosis
DVT deep venous thrombosis
ECG electrocardiograph
EF ejection fraction
ENT ear, nose and throat
ESC European Society of Cardiology
ESKD end-stage kidney disease
EWS early warning score
FAST Face Arm Speech Test
FBP full blood picture
FEV1 forced expiratory volume in one second
FFP fresh frozen plasma
FVC forced vital capacity
GABA gamma aminobutyric acid
GCS Glasgow Coma Scale
GFR glomerular filtration rate
GTN glyceryl trinitrate
Hb haemoglobin
HDU High Dependency Unit
HF heart failure
HR heart rate
ICP intracranial pressure
ICU Intensive Care Unit
IgE/IgM immunoglobulin E/immunoglobulin M
IM intramuscularly
INR international normalized ratio
IV intravenous
ISWP Intercollegiate Stroke Working Party
JVP jugular venous pressure
LABA long-acting beta-agonist
LAMA long-acting muscarinic antagonist
LDH lactate dehydrogenase
LFTs liver function tests
LMWH low molecular weight heparin
LV left ventricular
LVH left ventricular hypertrophy
LVSD left ventricular systolic dysfunction
MABP mean arterial blood pressure
MAP mean arterial pressure

MRC Medical Research Council
MRI magnetic resonance imaging
NHS National Health Service
NSAIDs non-steroidal anti-inflammatory drugs
NTproBNP N-terminal pro-brain natriuretic peptide
NYHA New York Heart Association
OGD oesophagogastroduodenoscopy
$PaCO_2$ partial pressure of carbon dioxide
PAI plasminogen-activator inhibitor
PaO_2 partial pressure of oxygen
PCI percutaneous coronary intervention
PE pulmonary embolism
PEFR peak expiratory flowrate
PICC peripherally inserted central catheter
PQRST Position and radiation, Quality, Relieving or exacerbating factors, Severity
    and Time
PT prothrombin time
PTH parathyroid hormone
PTT partial prothrombin time
RR respiratory rate
RSVP Reason, Story, Vital signs, Plan
SBAR Situation, Background, Assessment, Recommendation
SCr serum creatinine
SE status epilepticus
SIRS systemic inflammatory response syndrome
SNS sympathetic nervous system
SpO_2 saturation of peripheral oxygen
STEMI ST segment elevation myocardial infarction
TBSA total body surface area
TFTs thyroid function tests
TIA transient ischaemic attack
V/Q ventilation/perfusion
U&E urea and electrolytes
WCC white cell count

Karen Page and Aidín McKinney

It is widely acknowledged that many factors, including developments in technology and economic constraints, allied with continued demographic changes, have led to increasing patient acuity within the healthcare setting. The increasing complexity of medical and surgical care, coupled with a reduction in the length of in-patient stay, has increased the probability that a nurse will require skills to manage acutely ill patients in numerous settings (NICE 2007). However, as patient acuity has increased, evidence has emerged that the care of the acutely ill patient can be suboptimal (NPSA 2007). It is no surprise therefore that recognition and management of such patients are high on the National Health Service (NHS) agenda (NPSA 2007). The publication of the National Institute of Clinical Excellence (NICE 2007) guidance on the assessment and monitoring of the acutely ill patient highlights that this is an area which must be addressed both in the clinical area and in nurse education. NICE (2007) clearly stated that staff caring for patients in acute hospital settings should have competencies in monitoring, measurement, interpretation and prompt response to the acutely ill patient appropriate to the level of care they are providing. The Department of Health (2000) recognized that such patients are not only cared for in critical care or high dependency units but are often to be found in Accident and Emergency departments or in general medical and surgical wards. In these circumstances nurses are in an excellent position to identify acutely ill patients and possibly instigate actions to ensure a better outcome in the event of further deterioration (Gallagher et al. 2011). As a result of this, further emphasis is being placed on developing skills and knowledge with respect to the care of the acutely ill patient in undergraduate nursing curricula and post-registration training programmes.

Various initiatives have also been implemented across the NHS to address the issues that have been identified in respect to the failings in the early recognition and care of acutely ill or deteriorating patients. These include initiatives that focused on reviewing how acutely ill patients are assessed, the value of early warning scores and determining protocols to improve communication, in particular with regards to communicating in a timely and effective manner. These areas will be outlined briefly in this introductory chapter before identifying how this book may be a useful resource to enable nurses to further focus on these skills.

ASSESSMENT

Clinical signs of acute illness or deterioration in a patient's condition are often similar, whatever the underlying cause of the illness because they reflect deteriorating cardiovascular, respiratory and neurological function (Resuscitation Council (UK) 2011). The ABCDE approach to assessing the patient has therefore been designed to ensure that a rapid but thorough assessment is carried out. This approach which considers **A**irway, **B**reathing, **C**irculation, **D**isability and **E**xposure in turn is widely accepted as providing a uniform systematic approach which facilitates good multidisciplinary team working and the ability to identify and treat any problems in order of priority (Resuscitation Council (UK) 2011). This approach to assessment forms the basis of the evaluation of each of the patients which feature in the case studies in the following chapters and will be elaborated on in the relevant chapters.

EARLY WARNING SCORES (EWS)

Continued monitoring and reassessment of acutely ill patients are essential. Aggregated EWS have been developed and implemented in healthcare settings to facilitate the identification and continued monitoring of patients at risk (Prytherch et al. 2010). These early warning scoring systems (EWS) are also known as track and trigger systems. Both NCEPOD (2005) and NICE (2007) advocate that such systems should be used to monitor all patients in acute hospital settings. These systems have been designed to alert medical and nursing staff to the early signs of acute illness or the risk of deterioration in a patient's condition. There are a wide variety of systems in use; however, they all share the same principles. They all rely on the accurate measurement and recording of clinical observations in relation to selected physiological criteria. Each of the physiological criteria is allocated a score dependent on the patient presentation and all the scores are added together to give a final score. This should reflect the patient's condition and should trigger a response for contacting staff with competencies in the management of the deteriorating patient if required (NICE 2007). It is also essential, however, that staff have a sound understanding of normal and abnormal physiology to underpin the prompt recognition and assessment of the data collected (Clarke and Ketchell 2011).

COMMUNICATION

The Resuscitation Council (UK) (2011) suggests that communication problems contribute to 80 per cent of adverse incidents or near-miss reports in hospital. The ability to recognize physiological abnormalities and communicate with the wider clinical team to implement sound clinical decision-making is a key factor in the prevention of an impending adverse event. However, participants in a study involving experienced registered nurses conducted by Hartigan et al. (2010) highlighted that this continues to be a challenging area of practice for newly qualified staff. In view of this, protocols for summoning assistance to a deteriorating patient have been developed with the use of the SBAR or RSVP communication tools or treatment memory aids being implemented in many hospital trusts (Resuscitation Council (UK) 2011).

Check point: SBAR, RSVP

SBAR

S = Situation
B = Background

A = Assessment
R = Recommendation

RSVP

R = Reason
S = Story
V = Vital signs
P = Plan

These tools can assist members of the healthcare team to communicate their concerns concisely and effectively regarding the salient features of a patient's condition in any given situation. Moreover, this team has been extended to include the Critical Care Outreach Team which has led to the sharing of skills and expertise to collaborate and support the care of acutely ill ward-based patients whose condition is at risk of deterioration.

HOW THIS BOOK MAY BE OF VALUE TO THE PRACTITIONER

The aim of this book is to highlight how important aspects of the care of acutely ill patients should be embedded into your practice to prompt timely and effective interventions. A case study approach has been used to allow practitioners to contextualize their knowledge and understand the relevance of underpinning theory to clinical practice.

The various case studies seek to promote the following:

- recognition of the importance and understanding of the systematic assessment of the acutely ill patient;
- recognition of the relationship between the underlying pathophysiology and the presenting clinical symptoms;
- integration of knowledge of pathophysiology with the rationale for a range of clinical investigations and nursing care required by the acutely ill adult.

The patients cited in these case studies are entirely fictitious; however, the material is drawn from the experience of the various authors in collaboration with clinical colleagues and therefore represents situations which commonly occur in the clinical area. Each case study will select individual aspects of the care and management of the patient which are pertinent to the topic under discussion. However, it should be noted that the principles and practice of assessment and many of the interventions discussed within a particular subject area are relevant to other situations, e.g. provision of oxygen therapy, fluid resuscitation and pain management These case studies will therefore give the reader an opportunity to advance or refresh their knowledge of the practices and procedures used to recognize and respond to the early indicators of physiological changes and underpin clinical skills. Whether you are a nursing student or a more experienced practitioner either returning to practice or moving to a new area, this should enhance your confidence and ability to respond appropriately in acute care situations and facilitate sound clinical decision-making skills.

REFERENCES

Clarke, D. and Ketchell, A. (2011) *Nursing the Acutely Ill Adult: Priorities in Assessment and Management*. Basingstoke: Palgrave Macmillan.

Department of Health (2000) *Comprehensive Critical Care*. London: Department of Health.

Gallagher, P.J., Rice, B., Tierney, P., Page, K. and McKinney, A.A. (2011) An evaluation of a critical care course for undergraduate nursing students, *Nursing in Critical Care*, 16(5): 261.

Hartigan, I., Murphy, S., Flynn, A.V. and Walshe, N. (2010) Acute nursing episodes which challenge graduates' competence: perceptions of registered nurses, *Nurse Education in Practice*, 10: 291–7.

NCEPOD (National Confidential Enquiry into Patient Outcomes and Death) (2005) *An Acute Problem? A Report of the National Confidential Enquiry into Patient Outcome and Death*. London: NCEPOD.

NICE (National Institute for Health and Clinical Excellence) (2007) *Acutely Ill Patients in Hospital: Recognition of and Response to Acute Illness in Adults in Hospital*. Clinical Guideline 50. London: NICE.

NPSA (National Patient Safety Agency) (2007) *Safer Care for the Acutely Ill Patient: Learning from Serious Incidents*, Fifth Report from the Patient Safety Observatory. London: NPSA.

Prytherch, D.R., Smith, G.B., Schmidt, P.E. and Featherstone, P.I. (2010) ViEWS: towards a national early warning score for detecting adult in-patient deterioration, *Resuscitation*, 81(8): 932–7.

Resuscitation Council (UK) (2011) *Immediate Life Support*, 3rd edn. London: Resuscitation Council (UK).

PART 1
Cardiovascular System

Acute coronary syndrome
Patrick Gallagher

Case outline

Peter Brown is a 58-year-old gentleman who has experienced an episode of crushing central chest pain while at work. Peter works as a taxi driver and a colleague has taken him to the Accident and Emergency Department. On admission, Peter is sweaty, clammy, nauseated and short of breath. He is complaining of chest pain radiating to his left arm. This is Peter's first presentation to hospital and he has no relevant past medical history. Peter smokes approximately 20–30 cigarettes per day and takes alcohol at weekends only. Peter is anxious and is concerned that his wife and children are informed. He also states his father died suddenly following a heart attack a number of years ago. Peter is immediately triaged and taken to the resuscitation room. You are the receiving nurse.

Observations on admission include:

Respiratory rate: 18 breaths per minute
Oxygen saturations: 95%
Blood pressure: 150/90 mmHg
Pulse: 94 beats per minute
Temperature: 37°C.

On admission to hospital an electrocardiograph (ECG) has been undertaken. Peter has been diagnosed with an anterior ST segment elevation myocardial infarction (anterior STEMI). Blood samples have also been drawn for urea and electrolytes (U&E), full blood picture (FBP) and highly sensitive troponin T.

---

1 **Discuss Peter's immediate problems and explain these using your knowledge of pathophysiology.**

A On admission to Accident and Emergency (A&E), Peter will be assessed using the Manchester Triage system (Cooke and Jinks 1999) incorporating the ABCDE approach as per the Resuscitation Council (UK) (2011). The ABCDE assessment and management tool can be applied to all deteriorating or critically ill patients. It is recognized that approximately 30 per cent of people developing a myocardial infarction die before reaching hospital (Resuscitation Council (UK) 2011). Furthermore, Henderson (2010) states that in Europe the estimated incidence of acute coronary syndrome (ACS) lies between 1 in 80 and 1 in 170 of the population. While awareness of risk factors may reduce these figures, it is imperative that nursing staff are aware of the seriousness of ACS and the risk it poses to life. Effective and efficient assessment together with early treatment is at the heart of improving survival.

An ST elevation myocardial infarction is characterized by fissures or cracks in the atherosclerotic plaques of coronary arteries. As Henderson (2010) explains, plaque rupture triggers platelet aggregation and activation of the coagulation cascade. This results in coronary thrombosis and a resulting occlusion in the coronary artery. The size and pattern of the myocardial infarction are dependent on the location and extent of the occlusion.

Central crushing chest pain

When assessing the patient with a probable ACS, it is imperative to undertake a good history in relation to the patient's chest pain and presenting symptoms. It is notable that while chest pain is one of the main symptoms of ACS, it does not occur in 25 per cent of all cases (Naik et al. 2007). This is particularly common among patients with diabetes who may not sense pain due to peripheral neuropathy.

Chest pain arises due to myocardial ischaemia, and the coronary occlusion. As Woods et al. (2010) state, chest discomfort is related to an imbalance between oxygen supply and demand. Blood is essentially trying to 'push' its way past an obstruction. A myocardial infarction results when there is prolonged ischaemia, causing irreversible damage to the heart muscle. Part of the heart muscle is not receiving oxygenated blood due to an obstructed coronary artery. The lack of oxygenated blood contributes to the pain felt by Peter. Furthermore, the triggering of the inflammatory process, when there is myocardial injury together with the cellular change from aerobic to anerobic metabolism, causes an increase in the production of lactic acid. The inflammatory process together with the release of lactic acid causes swelling, oedema and increased pressure on nerve endings, resulting in chest pain.

Sweaty and clammy sensation

Significant coronary arterial occlusion will stimulate the sympathetic nervous system (SNS). This stimulation of the SNS will signal the release of adrenaline and noradrenaline from the adrenal medulla. Adrenaline release is rapid and will cause a tachycardia in an effort to maintain homeostasis. The release of adrenaline and noradrenaline also causes peripheral vasoconstriction due to their effects on alpha- and beta-adrenergic receptors (Karch 2008). The effect of these naturally occurring catechalomines is to make the skin feel sweaty, slightly cold and clammy. Furthermore, the release of catecholamines also heightens the state of anxiety by increasing the heart rate and blood pressure. Porth (2011) explains that the developing sympathetic stimulation gives rise to restlessness, tachycardia and a feeling of impending doom.

As the heart rate increases in an attempt to compensate for a reduction in contractility, there will be a corresponding rise in blood pressure. Peter's blood pressure rise can also be explained by the increase in catecholamine activity together with the pain experienced and the increased sympathetic activity. These compensatory activities cause a rise in blood pressure due to increased vasoconstriction, increased contractility and tachycardia. However, as the infarction develops, if left untreated, these compensatory activities will fail and may exacerbate the infarcted area of heart muscle. This is due to the increase in myocardial oxygen demand caused by the increase in heart rate. In other words, there is a tipping of the scale towards oxygen demand with an inability to supply the damaged myocardium as a result of coronary thrombosis.

Nausea

Nausea results from the stimulation of the medullary vomiting centre and often precedes vomiting (Porth 2007). The nausea a patient experiences with the development of an ACS may range from mild to severe and may indeed be accompanied with vomiting. Hypoxia can exert a direct effect on the vomiting centre and may account for the nausea and vomiting that occur in decreased cardiac output (Porth 2007). Nausea is frequently accompanied by autonomic nervous system manifestations such as excess salivation, vasoconstriction, sweating and pallor. The nausea Peter is experiencing seems to be explained by both the severity of the chest pain and the autonomic nervous system changes that take place due to the ACS.

Shortness of breath

Due to decreased blood flow to the affected myocardium, oxygen reserves are rapidly utilized. As a result, there is a change from aerobic to anaerobic metabolism, and, as Porth (2011) explains, this results in a striking loss of myocardial contractile function. The shortness of breath may be manifested by an increase in the respiratory rate together with a reduction in oxygen saturations. This increase in respirations may be due to the possible development of pulmonary oedema as the contractile function of the left ventricle deteriorates. Furthermore, due to the oxygen requirements of the myocardium, there is a need to increase the respiratory rate. While Peter is complaining of shortness of breath, his resulting observations dictate a patient who is compensating reasonably well with oxygen saturations of 95 per cent.

2 **Outline the nursing care that Peter should receive in relation to the problems identified.**

A Relief of pain may reduce the patient's anxiety and also halt the body's autonomic nervous system requirements. This in turn will have the effect of reducing cardiac workload (Antman 2008). The nurse should work in a calm, confident manner and explain that pain relief will be provided.

Obtaining a complete and detailed clinical history is essential when evaluating patients with suspected ischaemic coronary syndromes (Scirica 2010). Henderson (2010) explains that most patients with suspected ACS present with prolonged episodes of chest pain. Careful assessment of the patient's chest pain is essential. The pain could be assessed using the PQRST (Position, Quality, Radiation, Severity and Time) mnemonic as described by Cole et al. (2006). The position or location of cardiac pain is usually diffuse rather than localized to a single point. Pain with ACS could be precipitated by exercise and, as Henderson (2010) suggests, usually lasts longer than 20 minutes. The pain may radiate to the back, arms (particularly the left), neck, lower face and even upper abdomen (Naik et al. 2007). Furthermore, Naik et al. suggest the pain may be described as 'discomfort', 'tightness', 'heaviness' or 'gripping'.

Patients with suspected ACS complaining of chest pain should be given sublingual glyceryl trinitrate (GTN) and opioid analgesia to relieve symptoms of chest pain (Henderson 2010). GTN is a vasodilator and acts to increase blood supply to the heart muscle. Nitrates can also be given via the buccal route (Katzung 2004). When given sublingually, the nurse should continue to assess the patient's pain level, and as nitrates can lead to hypotension, the blood pressure should also be monitored. Porth (2011) explains that the vasodilating effects of nitrates decrease both preload (venous return) and afterload (arterial blood pressure). The net result of nitrates is to reduce myocardial oxygen consumption. Caution should be taken with patients who are hypotensive, or have any condition that limits cardiac output (Karch 2008). Furthermore, Karch (2008) explains that nitrates should be used with caution in patients with suspected cerebral haemorrhage (due to the possibility of increasing intracranial bleeding following relaxation of cerebral vessels). Aspirin 300 mg (dispersible) may also be given in the initial stage as it helps to reduce platelet aggregation and adhesion. Porth (2011) explains that aspirin is thought to promote reperfusion and reduce the likelihood of further thrombosis.

Although several analgesics can be used to treat the pain of ACS, the opiates, in particular morphine (or diamorphine), are usually the drug of choice (Smith and Whitwam 2006). Intravenous morphine (or diamorphine) should be titrated to control the patient's symptoms. However, as the Resuscitation Council (UK) (2011) explains, sedation and respiratory depression should be avoided. An antiemetic should also be given with the opiate analgesic in order to decrease levels of nausea. Tissues, mouthwash and an emesis bowl should also be provided.

Oxygen may also be used but, as the Resuscitation Council (UK) (2011) explains, nurses must remember to stay within the current guidelines, i.e. to keep the oxygen saturations between 94–98 per cent in patients without chronic obstructive pulmonary disease (COPD). For patients with COPD, the recommended level is between 88 and 92 per cent. However, the patient should be encouraged to sit in an upright position to help lung fields expand.

Check point: treatment memory aids

MOVE

M = Cardiac monitoring and regular monitoring of observations
O = Oxygen (if necessary)
V = Venous access and remember to take bloods
E = 12-lead ECG

MONA

M = Morphine or diamorphine
O = Oxygen (if necessary)
N = Nitrates
A = Aspirin

3   **Discuss the ECG that has been recorded with reference to the diagnosis.**

A   A 12-lead ECG should be recorded as a matter of urgency during the initial assessment (Figure 1.1). Porth (2011) recommends that as well as a 12-lead ECG, cardiac monitoring should be instigated immediately. While the importance of recording an ECG should not be underestimated, Morris and Whiteside (2008) suggest that it should be interpreted in the light of the clinical information. These authors explain that the ECG is not perfect and can be normal in the early stages of ST segment elevation myocardial infarction (STEMI).

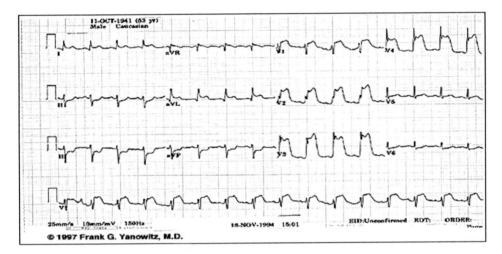

Figure 1.1 Acute anterior STEMI

Source: Frank G. Yanowitz, M.D., copyright 1997, available at: http://library.med.utah.edu/kw/ecg/mml/ecg_12lead028.html (accessed 28 April 2011).

> Peter's ECG shows ST segment elevation in leads V2, V3, V4 and to a lesser extent in V5. This is typical of an anterior ST elevation myocardial infarction (Hatchett and Thompson 2007). This ECG indicates that Peter should be treated urgently with a view to reperfusion therapy. Reperfusion therapy involves either thrombolytic therapy or being taken to the cardiac catheterization laboratory in order that a stent may be inserted in the culprit coronary artery.

4   **Discuss the relevance of taking a high-sensitivity troponin T**

A   A number of isoforms of the troponin complex exist. These are troponin I, T and C and they exist on the thin filament of myofibrils and regulate skeletal and cardiac muscle contraction (Henderson 2010). Troponins are sensitive and are markers of myocardial injury. Cardiac troponin begins to rise within 4 hours of the myocardial infarction and peaks between 24–48 hours. However, care should be taken with the interpretation of troponins. While a troponin rise does signify myocardial damage, it is not specific to ACS. Scirica (2010) explains that troponins can be elevated in patients with sepsis or pulmonary emboli, and while there is myocardial damage, it is not caused by ACS.

High-sensitivity troponins now offer greater sensitivity and earlier detection of myocardial injury. Melanson et al. (2007) report that 64 per cent of patients with initial negative troponin results actually had raised levels when using the high-sensitivity assay. While the use of highly sensitive troponins may lead to better diagnosis, caution should be exercised as Sabatine et al. (2009), in a small-scale study, found that exercise testing and transient stress-induced ischaemia were also associated with an elevated highly sensitive troponin rise. Troponin should therefore be used as an adjunct to both clinical assessment and the ECG interpretation in assisting the physician make a diagnosis.

Other bloods in particular potassium levels should also be observed. This is assayed on the urea and electrolytes (U&E) sample. The potassium should be kept within normal limits (usually 3.5–5.0 mmol/L). A potassium level outside these normal limits should be corrected in order to reduce the possibility of triggering cardiac arrhythmias (Resuscitation Council (UK) 2011). The full blood picture is taken to check for any signs such as a drop in haemoglobin, abnormal levels of platelets or white cells. A low level of haemoglobin can trigger chest pain and may warrant further investigation. Low levels of platelets may have implications for administering antiplatelet drugs and again warrants further investigation.

> The cardiologist has decided to take Peter to the cardiac catheterization laboratory (cath lab) to undergo a percutaneous coronary intervention (PCI) as opposed to giving him thrombolytic therapy. The cardiologist wants Peter to have clopidogrel 600 mg and aspirin 300 mg prior to transfer to the catheterization laboratory.

5 **Briefly discuss the benefits of PCI in comparison to thrombolytic therapy.**

A Randomized controlled trials suggest a significant benefit in favour of early invasive angiography together with the deployment of a stent. These trials (Mehta et al. 2005; NICE 2010) suggest an early invasive strategy is associated with a lower mortality and risk of recurrent ischaemia. The optimal timing for coronary angiography has not been elicited but for patients in a high risk group (early STEMI), then the benefits are greatest with significant reductions in risk of death if undertaken early.

6 **Discuss the modes of action of clopidogrel and aspirin and their use prior to PCI.**

A Both clopidogrel and aspirin are antiplatelet drugs and decrease the formation of the platelet plug. These drugs are used effectively in the treatment of cardiovascular diseases. Clopidogrel is known as an adenosine diphosphate (ADP) inhibitor and, as such, limits platelet adhesion and aggregation by stopping one pathway to platelet adhesion (Rang et al. 2003). Aspirin works by inhibiting the synthesis of a substance known as thromboxane A2 (Karch 2011). Patients requiring PCI are effectively 'loaded' with both drugs prior to the procedure. The dosage is determined by the cardiology consultant but is normally 300 mg for both drugs followed by aspirin 75 mg and clopidogrel 75 mg (Royal Pharmaceutical Society of Great Britain 2008).

Following Peter's transfer to the cath lab, he had a stent deployed to his left anterior descending coronary artery. Subsequently Peter made a full uncomplicated recovery and was discharged four days later.

Key points

- A 12-lead ECG should be recorded as a matter of urgency during the initial assessment. Troponins are sensitive and are markers of myocardial injury.
- Randomized controlled trials suggest a significant benefit in favour of early invasive angiography together with the deployment of a stent.

REFERENCES

Antman, E.M. (2008) ST elevation myocardial infarction: management, in P. Libby, R. Bonow and D.L. Mann (eds) *Braunwald's Heart Disease: A Textbook Of Cardiovascular Medicine*, 8th edn. Philadelphia, PA: Saunders Elsevier.

Cole, E., Lynch, A. and Cugnoni, H. (2006) Assessment of the patient with acute abdominal pain, *Nursing Standard*, 20(39): 67–75.

Cooke, M.W. and Jinks, S. (1999) Does the Manchester triage system detect the critically ill? *Journal of Accident and Emergency Medicine*, 16: 179–81.

Hatchett, R. and Thompson, D.R. (2007) *Cardiac Nursing: A Comprehensive Guide*, 2nd edn. Philadelphia, PA: Churchill Livingstone.

Henderson, R.A. (2010) Ischaemic heart disease: management of non-ST-elevation acute coronary syndrome, *Medicine*, 38(8): 424–30.

Karch, A.M. (2008) *Focus on Nursing Pharmacology*, 4th edn. London: Lippincott Williams and Wilkins.

Karch, A.M. (2011) *Focus on Nursing Pharmacology*, adapted by E. Sheader, T. Speake and C. Griffiths. London: Lippincott Williams and Wilkins.

Katzung, B.G. (2004) *Basic and Clinical Pharmacology*, 9th edn. Maidenhead: McGraw-Hill.

Mehta, S.R., Cannon, C.P. and Fox, K.A.A. (2005) Routine vs selective invasive strategies in patients with acute coronary syndromes: a collaborative meta-analysis of randomised trials, *Journal of American Medical Association*, 293: 2908–17.

Melanson, S.E., Morrow, D.A. and Jarolim, P. (2007) Earlier detection of myocardial injury in a preliminary evaluation using a new troponin I assay with improved sensitivity. *American Journal of Clinical Pathology*, 128: 282–6.

Morris, F. and Whiteside, M. (2008) Chest pain, *Medicine*, 32(2): 75–80.

Naik, H., Sabatine, M.S. and Lilly, L.S. (2007) *Pathophysiology of Heart Disease: A Collaborative Project of Medical Students and Faculty*, 4th edn. Philadelphia, PA: Lippincott Williams and Wilkins.

NICE (National Institute for Health and Clinical Excellence) (2010) Unstable angina and NSTEMI: the early management of unstable angina and non-ST-segment-elevation myocardial infarction. National Institute for Health and Clinical Excellence, available at: http://guidance.nice.org.uk/CG94/Guidance/pdf/English (accessed 21 April 2011).

Porth, C.M. (2007) *Essentials of Pathophysiology: Concepts of Altered Health States,* 2nd edn. London: Lippincott Williams and Wilkins.

Porth, C.M. (2011) *Essentials of Pathophysiology,* 3rd edn. London: Lippincott Williams and Wilkins.

Rang, H.P., Dale, M.M., Ritter, J.M. and Moore, P.K. (2003) *Pharmacology,* 5th edn. London: Churchill Livingstone.

Resuscitation Council (UK) (2011) *Advanced Life Support,* 6th edn. London: Resuscitation Council (UK).

Royal Pharmaceutical Society of Great Britain (2008) *British National Formulary.* London: Royal Pharmaceutical Society of Great Britain.

Sabatine, M.S., Morrow, D.A., de Lemos, J.A., Jarolim, P. and Braunwald, E. (2009) Detection of acute changes in circulating troponin in the setting of transient stress test-induced myocardial ischaemia using ultrasensitive assay: results from TIMI 35, *European Heart Journal,* 30: 162–9.

Scirica, B.M. (2010) Acute coronary syndrome emerging tools for diagnosis and risk assessment, *Journal of the American College of Cardiology,* 55(14): 1403–15.

Smith, S.W. and Whitwam, W. (2006) Acute coronary syndromes, *Emergency Medicine Clinics of North America,* 24: 53–89.

Woods, S.L., Sivarajan Froelicher, E.S., Underhill Motzer, S. and Bridges, E.J. (2010) *Cardiac Nursing,* 6th edn. Philadelphia, PA: Lippincott Williams and Wilkins.

Acute heart failure
Billie Joan Rice

Case outline

George, a 71-year-old retired electrician, presents to A&E complaining of increased dyspnoea on exertion and chronic fatigue. He has experienced increased dyspnoea over the past two years which has worsened over the past four weeks. He has had a recent respiratory tract infection and believed that the breathlessness may be due to this. He has started using three pillows at night due to night-time wheeze and coughing. He has noticed 'swelling' around his ankles over the past two weeks.

Past medical history:

MI at 58 years of age.
He suffers from hypertension and stable angina.

Current medication:

Aspirin 75 mg *mane*
Bendroflumethiazide 2.5 mg *mane*
Atenolol 50 mg *mane*
GTN spray as required
Simvastatin 40 mg *nocte*.

George has been a smoker for 30 years and has been unable to stop despite several attempts, although he has decreased his cigarette consumption from 20 cigarettes per day to 10. He enjoys a drink at his local social club and admits to drinking around 15 units/week of alcohol.

On examination, it is noted that George is breathless and there is increased work of his breathing. His extremities are cool to touch and have a blue 'tinge'.

1 **You suspect a diagnosis of chronic heart failure. Explain this term.**

A Chronic heart failure (CHF) is a complex clinical syndrome that can result from any structural or functional cardiac or non-cardiac disorder that impairs the ability of the heart to respond to physiological demands for cardiac output. Chronic heart failure is characterized by symptoms such as exertional breathlessness and fatigue, and signs of fluid retention as well as signs associated with the underlying cardiac disorder (SIGN 2007).

2   **Outline the triggers of CHF.**

A The commonest cause of heart failure is myocardial dysfunction, which is commonly systolic, i.e. there is reduced ventricular contraction. Around two-thirds of these cases result from coronary heart disease (CHD) and there is usually a past history of myocardial infarction. Worsening hypertension is another identifiable trigger. Others include:

- infections – commonly chest infections, myocarditis, pericarditis, endocarditis;
- valve disorders;
- cardiomyopathies;
- arrhythymias;
- decompensation of heart failure.

Co-morbidities, for example, diabetes, pulmonary disease, and non-adherence to treatment/ medication are identifiable triggers of CHF (SIGN 2007; Dickstein et al. 2008).

3   **Outline George's main clinical symptoms and explain why these occur, discussing the underlying pathophysiology.**

A George is presenting with increased dyspnoea, fatigue, increased work of breathing, ankle oedema, cough at night-time. These symptoms result from an underlying cardiac injury.
   Cardiac injury refers to examples of altered pathology leading to left ventricular (LV) dysfunction (Figure 2.1). Examples include myocardial infarction, hypertension, valve disorders, cardiomyopathies. This ultimately leads to pump failure which causes decreased stroke volume, decreased cardiac output and renal blood flow. As a result, the body's compensatory

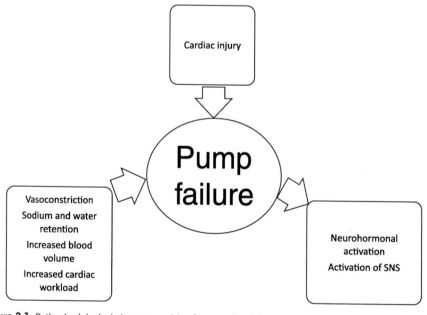

Figure 2.1 Pathophysiological changes resulting from cardiac injury

mechanisms are stimulated including the sympathetic nervous system (SNS). Both cardiac sympathetic tone and catecholamine (adrenaline and noradrenaline) levels are elevated during the late stages of most forms of heart failure. By direct stimulation of heart rate and cardiac contractility and by regulation of vascular tone, the sympathetic nervous system helps to maintain perfusion of the various organs, particularly the heart and brain.

The renin-angiotensin-aldosterone mechanism is stimulated due to the reduction in renal blood flow. With decreased renal blood flow, there is a progressive increase in renin secretion by the kidneys, along with parallel increases in circulating levels of angiotensin II. The increased concentration of angiotensin II contributes to a generalized and excessive vasoconstriction and provides a powerful stimulus for aldosterone production by the adrenal cortex. Aldosterone increases tubular reabsorption of sodium, with an accompanying increase in water retention. Angiotensin II also increases the level of anti-diuretic hormone (ADH), which serves as a vasoconstrictor and inhibitor of water excretion (Porth 2007).

The natriuretic peptide family consists of three peptides: (1) atrial natriuretic peptide (ANP); (2) brain natriuretic peptide (BNP); and (3) C-type natriuretic peptide (CNP). ANP, which is released from atrial cells in response to increased atrial stretch and pressure, produces rapid and transient natriuresis, diuresis and moderate loss of potassium in the urine. It also inhibits aldosterone and renin secretion, acts as an antagonist to angiotensin II, and inhibits the release of norepinephrine from presynaptic nerve terminals. BNP, so named because it was originally found in extracts of porcine brain, is stored mainly in the ventricular cells and is responsive to increased ventricular filling pressures. BNP has cardiovascular effects similar to those of ANP. Measurements of BNP are increasingly used to confirm the diagnosis of heart failure. It helps to evaluate the level of left ventricular compromise, estimate prognosis and predict future cardiac events (Porth 2007).

The endothelins, released from the endothelial cells throughout the circulation, are potent vasoconstrictors. Other actions of the endothelins include induction of vascular smooth muscle cell proliferation and myocyte hypertrophy.

The principal long-term mechanism by which the heart compensates for the increase in workload is the development of myocardial hypertrophy. Although ventricular hypertrophy may improve the work performance of the heart, it is also an important risk factor for subsequent cardiac morbidity and mortality. Inappropriate hypertrophy and remodelling can result in changes in structure (muscle mass, chamber dilation) and function (impaired systolic or diastolic function) that often lead to further pump dysfunction and haemodynamic overload (Porth 2007).

The outcome of all these changes is a collection of distressing symptoms, similar to George's, including dyspnoea, oedema and excessive fatigue.

4 **You will carry out a thorough assessment using the ABCDE assessment tool. In keeping with your suspected diagnosis, what might you expect to find?**

A **Check point: ABCDE assessment**

A + B = Airway and Breathing
C = Circulation
D = Disability
E = Exposure

Airway and breathing

- Airway and breathing will be assessed together as George is speaking in complete sentences, suggesting no airway obstruction.
- It is expected that the respiratory rate will be raised as the body attempts to compensate for a reduction in tissue perfusion.
- If pulmonary congestion is present, oxygen saturations will be low; otherwise SpO_2 (saturation of peripheral oxygen) levels can be normal in CHF patients (Allen and O'Connor 2007).
- George will be short of breath as the heart is unable to supply adequate oxygen to the tissues, thereby reducing exercise tolerance (Heart Failure Society of America 2006). Oxygen therapy is recommended in hypoxaemic patients with arterial oxygen saturations of <95% and should be instigated as early as possible (Dickstein et al. 2008; O'Driscoll et al. 2008).
- Auscultation of the chest should be performed to listen for basal crepitations.

Circulation

- Heart rate in CHF is frequently raised. Patients are tachycardic because the heart tries to compensate for a falling cardiac output by increasing the rate of contraction (Nicholson 2007).
- Hypertension can be both a cause and effect of CHF. Increased fluid volume increases both preload (the volume of blood returned to the heart) and afterload (the resistance against which the heart pumps) (Nicholson 2007).
- Jugular venous pressure (JVP) assessment is recommended as an initial assessment (Jevon and Ewen 2007; Dickstein et al. 2008). A raised JVP can be a good indicator of fluid overload as it correlates with right atrial pressure and increased preload (Whitlock 2010).
- If the top of the neck veins is more than 3 cm above the sternal angle, venous pressure is abnormally elevated. Elevated venous pressure reflects right ventricular failure (and is a late finding in left ventricular failure) (Woods et al. 2010).
- Assess the heart rhythm through cardiac monitoring and obtaining a 12-lead ECG. Many patients with heart failure have an underlying arrhythmia; in most cases, this is atrial fibrillation (AF) (Nicholson 2007). Some patients will have new onset AF, which their CHF may have precipitated. It can also be the cause of an acute episode of CHF (NCGC 2010).
- Auscultation of the heart may indicate a third heart sound, S3. This is an early diastolic low-pitched thudding sound that occurs after S2 (the aortic and pulmonary valve closure). It coincides with the phase of rapid ventricular filling (Kumar and Clark 2005). An S3 is caused by vibrations of the ventricles during ventricular filling which occurs when the mitral and tricuspid valves open. An abnormal S3 occurs when the left ventricle becomes less compliant or thickened (Lippincott Williams and Wilkins 2005) and is a common manifestation of left ventricular heart failure.
- Also obtain bloods – FBP, U&E, arterial blood gases (ABGs), troponin level, BNP levels, international normalized ratio (INR), thyroid function.

- Assess patient's fluid and salt intake and obtain patient's weight. Patients with CHF should be advised to avoid a salt intake of >6 g/day and healthcare professionals caring for patients with frequent decompensated heart failure should assess individual patients' fluid intake and use a tailored approach when giving fluid restriction advice (SIGN 2007). The European Society of Cardiology (ESC) (Dickstein et al. 2008) found evidence that restricting fluid intake while in stable CHF did not worsen or improve outcomes. Whitlock (2010) suggests that patients with signs of fluid overload can be advised to restrict fluid intake for the time it takes to off-load the excess fluid.
- The patient's weight can be a reliable indicator of fluid status. In particular, a picture of how much the weight has increased and how rapidly is important (Whitlock 2010).

Disability

Neurological status, specifically level of consciousness should be assessed using a tool such as AVPU or the Glasgow Coma Scale. Consciousness may be impaired due to cerebral hypoxia.

Exposure

- Assess the patient from head to toe, observing for signs of peripheral oedema commonly seen in the ankles but also in the sacrum and upper extremities. This can cause cellulitis, discomfort, sleep disturbance, altered body image and pressure sores.
- The patient can be assessed for functional capacity using the New York Heart Association (NYHA) functional classification (Table 2.1) (NYHA 1994). This scale is widely used to categorize the patient's condition and can be used to guide patient management.

Table 2.1 New York Heart Association functional classification scale

Class	Symptoms
I	Patients with cardiac disease but without resulting limitation of physical activity. Ordinary physical activity does not cause undue fatigue, palpitation, dyspnea or anginal pain
II	Patients with cardiac disease resulting in slight limitation of physical activity. They are comfortable at rest. Ordinary physical activity results in fatigue, palpitation, dyspnea or anginal pain
III	Patients with cardiac disease resulting in marked limitation of physical activity. They are comfortable at rest. Less than normal activity causes fatigue, palpitation, dyspnea or anginal pain
IV	Patients with cardiac disease resulting in inability to carry out any physical activity without discomfort. Symptoms of heart failure or the anginal syndrome may be present even at rest. If any physical activity is undertaken, discomfort increases

Source: NYHA, 1994

5 **Following your assessment, decide what investigations should be arranged for George and explain what you might find in CHF.**

A
- *Chest X-ray:* To show extent of pulmonary congestion and heart size, any pleural effusions or infection. To exclude other causes of shortness of breath.
- *12-lead ECG:* To identify pathological Q waves, left bundle branch block, left ventricular hypertrophy, arrhythmias – AF, non-specific ST and/or T wave changes. Q waves indicate previous myocardial infarction, left ventricular hypertrophy (LVH) is seen in hypertension and aortic valve disease and it is important to exclude atrial fibrillation (SIGN 2007).
- *Echocardiogram:* The gold standard investigation in terms of assessing the level of cardiac dysfunction and in identifying potential causes of HF such as valve and left ventricular dysfunction (NCGC 2010). The extent of left ventricular systolic dysfunction (LVSD) can be measured during echocardiograph by the ejection fraction (EF) (Chen et al. 2006). AHA (2010) states that a normal EF should be between 55% and 70% and that even with a normal EF, HF can still be present.

6 **Explain the key blood tests required in CHF.**

A
- *Full blood count (FBC):* FBC determines haemoglobin (Hb) levels, which is important as 15–55% of CHF patients have underlying anaemia (Westenbrink et al. 2007). Anaemia can be caused by reduced renal perfusion resulting in reduced erythropoietin production.
- A *high white cell count* can indicate infection (Skinner 2003).
- *C-reactive protein (CRP):* If the white cells are raised and CRP is elevated, this should prompt urgent septic screening, including sputum, urine samples, blood cultures and swabs of any wounds (Whitlock 2010).
- *Renal profile:* Urea and electrolytes. A renal profile will show how efficiently the kidneys are functioning and will provide an indication of the extent of renal perfusion, fluid volume status and also serum levels of potassium, sodium and creatinine. Rising creatinine and urea levels are an indication of worsening renal function and/or reduced renal perfusion, but high levels can be seen when the patient has been over-diuresed or is dehydrated and there is a resulting element of haemoconcentration (Whitlock 2010).
- *Glomerular filtration rate (GFR):* A faster, more accurate indicator of renal perfusion/function as a low perfusion can result in acute kidney injury with a resulting raised creatinine (Byrne and Murphy 2008).
- *International normalized ratio (INR):* Important to obtain in heart failure patients with atrial fibrillation who are taking warfarin.
- *Arterial blood gases (ABGs):* A more reliable evaluation of oxygenation of the patient and their acid–base balance and respiratory function.
- *Troponin levels:* To confirm if the patient has experienced an acute coronary event and will show extent of myocardial injury. Troponin levels should be taken in all patients presenting with chest pain and/or ECG changes and should be repeated 12 hours later to obtain a peak level (Whitlock 2010).
- *B-type natriuretic peptide (BNP) or N-terminal pro-brain natriuretic peptide (NTproBNP):* These are peptide hormones produced in the heart by the breakdown of a precursor protein (pro-BNP). BNP causes natriuresis, diuresis, vasodilation and muscle relaxation; NT-proBNP is inactive.

- Plasma BNP and NTproBNP concentrations are raised in patients with heart failure and the concentrations tend to rise with NYHA functional class (SIGN 2007) (see Table 2.1).
- BNP and NT proBNP are suitable for widespread use as a screening test in patients with suspected chronic heart failure, assuming appropriate quality control of the assay and selection of appropriate cut-off values for the patients tested. BNP levels fall after commencing therapy for CHF, e.g. diuretics, so the sensitivity is lower in patients who have already commenced treatment (SIGN 2007).
- BNP levels and proBNP levels and/or an electrocardiogram should be recorded to indicate the need for echocardiography in patients with suspected heart failure (SIGN 2007).
- *Liver function tests (LFTs).*
- *Thyroid function tests (TFTs)*: LFTs and TFTs should be checked as these may be deranged in HF due to hepatic congestion and drug toxicity (Davies et al. 2006).

> George's blood results show potassium 3.7 mmol/L (normal range 3.5–5.0 mmol/L) and serum creatinine 100 micromol/L (normal range 70–110 micromol/L). His ECG shows left bundle branch block. His chest X-ray shows mild cardiac enlargement. George is admitted to a medical ward to monitor his fluid/oedema and respiratory status. During his admission the bendroflumethiazide 2.5 mg is changed to furosemide 40 mg daily and his U&E checked daily.

7   **Explain why furosemide would be the drug of choice at this stage.**

A   Furosemide is a loop diuretic and acts upon the ascending limb of the loop of Henle. It inhibits the reabsorption of sodium and chloride ions from the loop into the interstitial fluid. The result of this is that the interstitial fluid becomes relatively hypotonic. A hypotonic interstitial fluid will result in a diuresis (Galbraith et al. 1999).

In the majority of heart failure patients, fluid retention occurs, causing ankle oedema, pulmonary oedema or both, contributing to the symptom of dyspnoea. Diuretic treatment relieves oedema and dyspnoea.

A major problem of the loop diuretic is electrolyte loss from the body. Potassium and sodium are the main ions affected. Potassium loss can lead to hypokalaemia, which can result in cardiac arrhythmias and even death. Monitoring a patient's U&E levels while taking furosemide is therefore important. Furosemide would be chosen at this stage, to relieve George's symptoms of dyspnoea and oedema.

> During his stay George has echocardiography performed which shows left ventricular systolic dysfunction (LVSD) and a left ventricular ejection fraction of 45%.

8   **Based on this finding, what changes, if any, should be made to George's medication and why?**

A   The results from the echocardiogram confirm that George has CHF. The aim of therapy in HF is to improve life expectancy and quality of life. Initial action to be taken because of the diagnosis of CHF is:

- Recheck blood electrolytes (especially potassium), urea, creatinine and BP.
- Add in an angiotensin-converting enzyme inhibitor (ACEI).

Choose from the following list:

> Captopril: starting dose = 6.25 mg TID, target dose 50 mg TID.
> Enalapril: starting dose = 2.5 mg twice daily, target dose 10–20 mg twice daily.
> Lisinopril: starting dose = 2.5–5 mg once daily, target dose 5 mg twice daily or 10 mg once daily.
> Ramipril: 2.5 mg once daily, target dose 5 mg twice daily or 10 mg once daily.
>
> (SIGN 2007)

George was commenced on ramipril 2.5 mg once daily. He was advised to double the dose at not less than two-weekly intervals until the target dose or maximum tolerated dose is achieved.

Recheck the electrolytes and BP after each dose titration. Good practice is to advise George to take the first dose of ACEI at night and to stop diuretics for 24 hours before hand to minimize the risk of first-dose hypotension. Aim for the targeted dose, or failing that, the highest tolerated dose (SIGN 2007).

George was initially prescribed a beta-blocker – atenolol. It was decided to change the atenolol to bisoprolol 1.25 mg once daily with a target dose of 10 mg once daily.

---

9   **Explain the use of beta-blockers in the management of CHF.**

A There is consistent evidence for positive benefits from beta-blockers in patients with heart failure, with the risk of mortality from cardiovascular causes reduced by 29% and all cause mortality reduced by 23%. Benefits were seen with beta-blockers with different pharmacological properties, whether B1 selective (bisoprolol, metoprolol, nebivolol) or non-selective (carvedilol).

Beta-blockers produce benefit in the medium to long term. In the short term, they can produce decompensation with worsening of heart failure and hypotension (SIGN 2007). Beta-blockers decrease the rate and force of contraction of the heart, decrease cardiac output and reduce blood pressure.

All patients with heart failure due to left systolic dysfunction of all NYHA functional classes should be started on beta-blocker therapy as soon as their condition is stable (unless contraindicated by a history of asthma, heart block or symptomatic hypotension).

Bisoprolol, carvedilol or nebivolol should be the beta-blocker of first choice for the treatment of patients with chronic heart failure due to left ventricular systolic dysfunction (SIGN 2007).

George is referred to the heart failure clinic and specialist heart failure nurse to assist in monitoring his condition.

10 **What education and lifestyle advice should the heart failure nurse offer George about CHF, prior to discharge?**

A She should do the following:

- Provide education about the condition of CHF.
- Explain the purpose of each prescribed medication, including timescale of expected benefits, and common side effects to support concordance.
- Strongly advise George not to smoke and offer support for smoking cessation.
- Give advice and support for weight management.
- Advise daily weighing at a set time every day. Report to the GP any noticeable weight gain over a short period. SIGN (2007) guidelines advise that patients should report weight gains of more than 1.5–2 kg in 2 days.
- Give dietary advice to avoid a salt intake of >6 g/day (approximately 1.5 teaspoons).
- Advise that the sodium content on food labels can be converted into salt content by multiplying by 2.5. Patients should be educated in the salt content of common foods.
- Advise George to continue to exercise. Walking is safe and reduces cardiopulmonary morbidity, and is good for mental health. Advise him to aim for at least a 30-minute walk every day. Both aerobic exercise such as walking and restive exercise such as weight training can improve symptoms, exercise performance and quality of life.

George may be concerned about any possible effect on his sex life either from the condition of CHF or from the drug treatments, but may be embarrassed to raise this. Guidelines advise that healthcare professionals should be prepared to broach subjects such as sexual activity with patients, as these are unlikely to be raised by the patient.

HF guidelines vary in their recommendations regarding alcohol, but all agree that alcohol is a myocardial depressant and patients with heart failure should refrain from excessive alcohol consumption. European guidelines recommend a limit of 1 or 2 units as a maximum per day. George's current alcohol intake of 15 units per week is slightly higher than this, but is under the national recommended maximum of 21 units per week for men, so is within acceptable limits. The walk to his social club and continued social contact will benefit George, but this level of alcohol intake should not be exceeded. SIGN (2007) recommend that all patients with heart failure should be advised to refrain from excessive alcohol consumption. When the aetiology of heart failure is alcohol-related, patients should be strongly encouraged to stop drinking alcohol.

Screen for depression in heart failure patients. Depression is common with CHF and is associated with an increased risk of mortality in some (SIGN 2007).

Key points

- CHF is a complex syndrome that impairs the ability of the heart to respond to increased demands for cardiac output.
- Treatment includes a range of drugs including diuretics, ACE inhibitors and beta-blockers.
- Referral to a heart failure nurse specialist can assist in monitoring the patient's condition.

REFERENCES

AHA (American Heart Association) (2010) *Ejection Fraction Heart Failure Measurement.* Available at: http://tinyurl.com/28hhgrz (accessed 5 December 2010).

Allen, L.A. and O'Connor, C.M. (2007) Management of acute decompensated heart failure, *Canadian Medical Association Journal*, 176: 797–805.

Byrne, G. and Murphy, F. (2008) Acute kidney injury and its impact on the cardiac patient, *British Journal of Cardiac Nursing*, 3(9): 416–22.

Chen, A.A., Wood, M.J., Krauser, D.G. et al. (2006) NT-pro BNP levels, echocardiographic findings and outcomes in breathless patients results from the ProBNP Investigation of Dyspnoea in the Emergency Department (PRIDE) echocardiographic substudy, *European Heart Journal*, 27: 839–45.

Davies, R.C., Davies, M.K. and Lip, G.Y.H. (2006) *ABC of Heart Failure*, 2nd edn. London: BMJ Publishing.

Dickstein, K., Cohen-Solal, A., Filippatos, G., McMurray, J.J.V. and All Task Force Members (2008) *ESC Guidelines for the Diagnosis and Treatment of Acute and Chronic Heart Failure 2008.* The Task Force for the Diagnosis and Treatment of Acute and Chronic Heart Failure 2008 of the European Society of Cardiology, developed in collaboration with the Heart Failure Association of the ESC (HFA) and endorsed by the European Society of Intensive Care Medicine (ESICM), *European Heart Journal*, 29: 2388–442.

Galbraith, A., Bullock, S., Manias, E., Hunt, B. and Richards, A. (1999) *Fundamentals of Pharmacology.* Harlow: Pearson Prentice Hall.

Heart Failure Society of America (2006) Development and implementation of a comprehensive heart failure practice guideline, *Journal of Cardiac Failure*, 12(1): e3–e103.

Jevon, P. and Ewens, B. (2007) *Monitoring the Critically Ill Patient*, 2nd edn. Oxford: Blackwell Science.

Kumar, P. and Clark, M. (2005) *Clinical Medicine*, 6th edn. Edinburgh: Elsevier Saunders.

Lippincott Williams and Wilkins (2005) *Heart Sounds Made Incredibly Easy.* Philadelphia, PA: Lippincott Williams and Wilkins.

NCGC (National Clinical Guideline Centre for Acute and Chronic Conditions) (2010) *Chronic Heart Failure: National Clinical Guideline for Diagnosis and Management in Primary and Secondary Care* (full version of NICE CG108). Available at: http://guidance.nice.org.uk/CG108 (accessed 5 December 2011).

Nicholson, C. (2007) *Heart Failure: A Clinical Nursing Handbook.* Chichester: Wiley and Sons Ltd.

NYHA (New York Heart Association) (1994) *Nomenclature and Criteria for Diagnosis of Diseases of the Heart and Great Vessels*, 9th edn. Boston: Little Brown & Co.

O'Driscoll, B., Howard, L., Davison, A. for the British Thoracic Society (2008) Guideline for emergency oxygen use in adult patients. Available at: http://tinyurl.com/2e9c7uv (accessed 5 December 2011).

Porth, C.M. (2007) *Essentials of Pathophysiology*, 2nd edn. Philadelphia, PA: Lippincott Williams and Wilkins.

SIGN (Scottish Intercollegiate Guidelines Network) (2007) *Management of Chronic Heart Failure: A National Clinical Guideline*. Edinburgh: Scottish Intercollegiate Network.

Skinner, S. (2003) *Understanding Clinical Investigations: A Quick Reference Manual*. London: Baillière Tindall.

Westenbrink, B.D., Visser, F.W., Voors, A.A., et al. (2007) Anaemia in chronic heart failure is not only related to impaired renal perfusion and blunted erythropoietin production, but to fluid retention as well, *European Heart Journal*, 28: 166–71.

Whitlock, A. (2010) Acute heart failure: patient assessment and management, *British Journal of Cardiac Nursing*, 5(11): 516–25.

Woods, S.L., Svarajan Froelicher, E.S., Underhill Motzer, S. and Bridges, E.J. (2010) *Cardiac Nursing*. Philadelphia, PA: Wolters Kluwer/Lippincott Williams and Wilkins.

PART 2
Respiratory System

CASE STUDY 3
Acute exacerbation of asthma
Karen Page

Case outline

Fiona is a 29-year-old lady with a history of asthma though this is normally well controlled with the use of regular inhalers. However, a few days ago she developed a mild cold and subsequently began to experience increasing shortness of breath with a reduction in her peak expiratory flow rate (PEFR). Today she has become extremely short of breath despite taking increased doses of her regular inhaler and has arrived at the A&E unit accompanied by her husband. She is dyspnoeic, anxious, distressed, pale and clammy with evidence of increased work of breathing. Consequently it is apparent that Fiona will need immediate treatment so she is admitted for further assessment and management.

1 **Identify and provide a rationale for the potential findings of Fiona's assessment on admission to the department.**

A All patients presenting with a severe dyspnoea require a thorough and objective assessment of the severity of their condition using a rapid ABCDE approach to indicate the correct management strategies (Stanley and Tunicliffe 2008).

HISTORY TAKING

If the patient's condition permits, a brief history can be obtained as part of a clinical examination. A brief history can be completed by asking a few questions to determine the patient's normal asthma condition and assess the severity of the present acute attack. Where possible, closed questions should be used and the patient should not be rushed as they will find talking difficult in this situation (Kennedy 2007). These brief questions will, however, allow the nurse to assess the patient's mental state and whether they are orientated to time and place as patients who are hypoxic can become confused. If the patient is unable to speak in full sentences, the nurse should curtail the history taking. Nevertheless, the amount of inhaled β-agonist self-administered prior to admission should be ascertained as this is a good marker of the severity of the acute attack and risk of a poor outcome (Aldington and Beasley 2007). Information on the patient's past medical history, previous admissions or attendances at Accident and Emergency and current treatments are also crucial factors in completing the

Table 3.1 The ABCDE procedure in the case of asthma

Potential clinical findings	Rationale
Airway General appearance	The general appearance of any patient is often a useful guide to the severity of their condition; however, it is important to note that a patient may be experiencing a serious acute asthma attack with severe airflow obstruction while still appearing deceptively well (Stanley and Tunicliffe 2008)
Difficulty in talking or completing sentences	If the patient can speak in sentences, the airway is not significantly impaired (Resuscitation Council (UK) 2011). In acute severe asthma, however, a patient may be unable to speak in full sentences because of the need to pause for breath. This inability to speak in full sentences is clinically significant and in asthma is considered a sign of a severe or life-threatening exacerbation (BTS and SIGN 2011)
Breathing Increased respiratory rate	The respiratory rate should be ascertained by counting the number of breaths for a full minute to ensure an accurate result. Evidence of tachypnoea or a respiratory rate ≥ 25 breaths per minute is a useful simple indicator of severe asthma (BTS and SIGN 2011). In addition to the respiratory rate, the breathing pattern should be noted including the regularity and depth of respirations (Kennedy 2007). Moreover, the symmetry of chest expansion should also be noted to exclude evidence of pneumothorax
Use of accessory muscles to assist the work of breathing	The use of the accessory muscles of respiration indicates increased respiratory effort on the part of the patient. The main respiratory muscles are the diaphragm and intercostal muscles; however, when breathing becomes laboured, patients use accessory muscles – scalene and sternocleidomastoids to make breathing easier. This requires substantial effort and uses valuable energy which may lead to exhaustion if prolonged. Pursed lips and nasal flaring are also indicators of laboured breathing (Hunter and Rawlings-Anderson 2008)
Altered posture	A patient's posture can often indicate the level of breathing difficulty that they are experiencing. Patients with increased work of breathing prefer to sit as upright as possible and avoid lying flat as this will worsen their breathing difficulties. Patients with impaired respiratory function often adopt a tripod position. This involves the patient resting their arms on their knees, arms of a chair or a bedside table. This is a way of splinting the lungs to allow maximum expansion (Kennedy 2007)

Presence of wheeze	An obvious expiratory wheeze is usually present in a patient with asthma although this may also be present later on inspiration. Narrowing of the airways and subsequent increase in airway resistance produce a wheeze. As the severity of asthma increases, breath sounds decrease and diminish due to airway closure. Note that the absence of wheeze, or 'quiet chest' is associated with a life-threatening degree of asthma (Marotta et al. 2010)
Has the patient got a cough?	The patient may have a cough with or without the production of mucus. At times the mucus is so tightly wedged in the narrowed airways that despite coughing, the patient is unable to expectorate this (Smeltzer et al. 2008)
Altered SpO$_2$ levels	Measurements of oxygen saturation by pulse oximetry should be undertaken in all patients with severe asthma presenting to hospital (Aldington and Beasley 2007).
Alteration of blood gas parameters	Analysis of blood gases can be reserved for those patients with oxygen saturations on room air of <92% or those who do not respond to initial treatment. Changes in blood gas measurements can indicate the severity of an acute asthma attack
Decreased lung function test results	Spirometry with measurement of forced expiratory volume (FEV1) is a useful measure of lung function and assessment of airflow obstruction. FEV1 is the maximum volume of air exhaled during the first second of a forced expiration. If this is not available, a peak flow reading is a helpful measure in detecting the severity of asthma and the patient's response to therapy. PEFR provides a simple and effective measure of airway function in the patient with asthma. Peak expiratory flow may decrease to 33–50% of the patient's known or predicted best measurement in acute severe asthma. A breathless patient may, however, be unable to complete ANY lung function assessment in an acute asthma attack
Chest X-ray results	A chest X-ray is not routinely recommended in an acute severe asthma attack unless the patient fails to respond to treatment, an alternative diagnosis is suspected such as pneumonia or pneumothorax, or ventilation is required (BTS and SIGN 2011)
Circulation Colour – cyanosis	Central cyanosis (a bluish discoloration of the skin or mucous membranes) is a late sign and indicates the presence of severe hypoxia. It is usually undetectable until oxygen saturations drop below 85% (Kennedy 2007)
Cool clammy skin	The patient may exhibit signs of diaphoresis due to anxiety, the increased work of breathing and the initiation of the sympathetic nervous system response mediated via the release of epinephrine (adrenaline)

(Continued overleaf)

Table 3.1 (*Continued*)

Potential clinical findings	Rationale
Pulse	Increasing pulse rate has a close correlation with worsening asthma severity and it is incorrect to assume that the tachycardia is simply due to β-agonist treatment (Aldington and Beasley 2007)
Blood pressure	Pulses parodoxus may be present – a physiological swing in systolic blood pressure which accompanies respiration. This may be demonstrated by a swing of more than 12 mmHg during inspiration. First appears when FEV1 has fallen to below 50%
Full blood picture and urea and electrolyte alterations	Full blood picture may indicate a raised white cell count in the presence of infection or the presence of eosinophilia and elevated serum immunoglobulin E (IgE) associated with allergy (Smeltzer et al. 2008). Hypokalaemia caused primarily by high dose β agonist therapy is not uncommon in severe asthma and may require potassium supplementation (Aldington and Beasley 2007)
Possible cardiac arrhythmias	ECG is a useful tool to detect the presence of possible arrhythmias which may be associated with the presence of electrolyte disturbances
Increased temperature	Temperature may be raised in the presence of infection or due to the increased work of breathing
Disability Decreased AVPU response	Altered level of response such as confusion or decreasing level of consciousness may indicate the presence of hypoxia
Exposure	No evidence of rashes, bleeding or bruising

assessment. However, to avoid the patient having to provide all the information at this time, previous existing medical notes should be accessed as soon as possible. Some of this information may often be obtained from relatives and since Fiona was accompanied by her husband, he was able to provide useful background details to staff regarding his wife. This also assists relatives in feeling involved in the care of the patient and allows interaction between the staff and relatives which is vital in supporting both the patient and family at a very anxious time for them all. The main priority though is to quickly identify those patients who are at increased risk of serious morbidity and mortality from asthma so an initial rapid clinical assessment is essential.

An assessment of this patient revealed the following information: Fiona was unable to speak in complete sentences, gasping for breath every few words, although she was orientated to time and place. Clinical observations included:

BP: 130/80 mmHg
Pulse: 128 beats per minute
Respirations: 36 breaths per minute and laboured
Temperature: 37.6°C
SpO_2: 88%.

A marked expiratory wheeze was evident with the use of accessory muscles to assist the work of breathing. Fiona was unable at this point to complete a peak flow reading. Blood gas analysis demonstrated PaO_2 (partial pressure of arterial oxygen) 8.0 kPa, $PaCO_2$ (partial pressure of arterial carbon dioxide) 5.0 kPa, pH 7.43.

2   **Why is blood gas analysis a useful indicator of the severity of an acute asthma attack?**

A   In the early stages of an acute asthmatic episode the patient will exhibit hypoxaemia without CO_2 retention. Hypoxaemia further increases hyperventilation through stimulation of the respiratory centre, causing $PaCO_2$ to decrease and pH to increase, causing respiratory alkalosis. Respiratory alkalosis is defined as a pH greater than 7.45 with a $PaCO_2$ less than 34 mmHg (4.5 kPa). Patients who have respiratory alkalosis have dramatically increased work of breathing and must be monitored closely for respiratory muscle fatigue.

As the obstruction becomes more severe, the number of alveoli which are inadequately ventilated and perfused increases, causing further alterations in the blood gases. As expiratory air flow obstruction increases, trapping airflow in the lungs, the lungs and thorax become hyperexpanded putting the respiratory muscles at a mechanical disadvantage. When the respiratory muscle becomes exhausted, CO_2 retention and respiratory acidosis ensue. A raised $PaCO_2 \geq 6$ kPa indicates the presence of respiratory acidosis which signals respiratory failure. While this is not often seen in an acute asthma attack, it indicates the presence of life-threatening asthma which requires urgent intervention (Rees et al. 2010).

Check point: asthma attack

The presence of any one of the following clinical features is considered to be associated with an acute severe asthma attack (BSG and SIGN 2011):

- Respiratory rate ≥ 25 breaths per minute.
- Breathlessness and inability to complete sentences.
- Pulse rate ≥ 110 beats per minute.
- PEFR 33–50% predicted normal value or patient's personal best value.

3   **Briefly outline the main underlying pathological changes found in asthma and explain why these lead to the increased respiratory rate and breathlessness experienced by Fiona.**

A   The basic underlying pathology in asthma is reversible and causes diffuse airway inflammation (Porth 2011). Exposure to an allergen or irritant substance initiates a

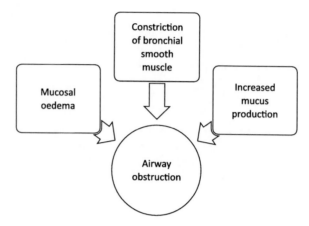

Figure 3.1 Events leading to airway obstruction in asthma

cascade of inflammatory events (Figure 3.1) which leads to airway obstruction as a result of:

1 increased capillary permeability leading to oedema of the membranes that line the airways which reduces the airway diameter;
2 contraction of the bronchial smooth muscle that encircles the airways causing further narrowing;
3 increased mucus production which may entirely plug the bronchi.

This leads to prolonged expiration and increased work of breathing in an acute asthma attack.

Respiratory rate ≥25 breaths per minute

Bronchoconstriction and mucus plugging cause incomplete exhalation, leading to air trapping in the lung which causes end expiratory lung volume to increase. Hyperventilation is triggered by lung receptors responding to the increased lung volume. The continued air trapping leads to variable and uneven ventilation perfusion ratios within different lung segments. The under-ventilated lung segments contribute poorly oxygenated blood to the arterial circulation, resulting in ventilation–perfusion mismatch and hypoxaemia (Marotta et al. 2010). Respiratory rate further increases to compensate for hypoxaemia due to reduced alveolar ventilation.

Breathlessness and inability to complete sentences

Hyperinflation of the lung puts respiratory muscles at a mechanical disadvantage and increases the work of breathing (Porth 2011). The increased effort of breathing, together with the pronounced increase in respiratory rate, leads the patient to experience breathlessness and difficulty in speaking.

4 **Discuss the rationale underpinning the essential management strategies required to treat Fiona's acute asthma attack and highlight the key related nursing interventions.**

A Aggressive treatment along with close observation must be initiated promptly during an acute asthma exacerbation to avoid rapid deterioration (Marotta et al. 2010).

Oxygen therapy

Fiona was prescribed supplemental oxygen to maintain an SpO_2 level of 94–98% (BTS and SIGN 2011).

Nursing interventions

- Explain the need for oxygen therapy and administer high flow oxygen as prescribed by the registered practitioner.
- Humidified oxygen may be required to assist in maintaining the moisture of the oral mucosa and secretions.
- Record pulse oximetry regularly and report any deterioration immediately.
- Ensure arterial blood gas measurements are obtained as required directing oxygen therapy if SpO_2 ≤92%.
- Patients with increased work of breathing prefer to sit as upright as possible to facilitate the work of breathing. Provide a bedside table and pillows to facilitate best use of their accessory muscles and maximize chest expansion.
- Ensure resuscitation equipment is readily available in the event of rapid respiratory deterioration.

Pharmacological therapy

Fiona was prescribed salbutamol 5 mg via nebuliser to be repeated if necessary at 20–30 minute intervals, and ipratropium bromide 0.5 mg via nebuliser repeated if necessary at 20–30 minute intervals.

Selective beta$_2$-adrenoceptor agonists such as salbutamol are the mainstay of short-acting bronchodilator therapy. Smooth muscle is an important component of the structure of the tracheobronchial tree. The smooth muscle fibres are arranged along the length of this structure in a double helical or spiral pattern and this formation profoundly influences the diameter and lumen of the airways. Consequently, the effect of muscle contraction reduces the diameter and length of the bronchial airway. Furthermore, the airway is innervated by the autonomic nervous system. The balance maintained between sympathetic and parasympathetic stimuli during rest influences the tone of the bronchial smooth muscle. The release of acetylcholine activates muscarinic receptors during stimulation of the parasympathetic system which results in *bronchoconstriction* causing narrowing of the bronchial airway. In contrast, the sympathetic nervous system affects adrenergic receptors. Most of the adrenergic receptors present in the bronchial smooth muscle are β_2 receptors that are stimulated mainly by epinephrine released from the adrenal medulla. Their action on the β_2 receptor sites produces *bronchodilation* by means of smooth muscle relaxation which improves ventilation to the lungs (McKenry et al. 2006).

Short-acting β_2-agonist drugs

β_2-agonists are sympathomimetic drugs that mimic the effects of the sympathetic nervous system. One of the actions of the sympathetic nervous system is dilation of the bronchi with increased rate and depth of respiration. Salbutamol, a sympathomimetic drug, possesses a relatively selective specificity for the β_2-adrenergic receptors in the lungs and therefore is less likely to cause unwanted cardiovascular side effects. The adverse effects include increased cardiac output, tachycardia, and arrhythmia. β_2-adrenoceptor agonists act specifically on the bronchial smooth muscle to cause smooth muscle relaxation, thus relieving bronchospasm and decreasing airway resistance during an asthma attack (McKenry et al. 2006). In patients with severe asthma that is poorly responsive to an initial bolus dose of β_2-agonist, continuous nebulisation with an appropriate nebuliser may be considered. In hospital, nebulised β_2-agonist bronchodilator therapy should be driven by oxygen (BTS and SIGN 2011).

Antimuscarinics are used as bronchodilators because of their antagonism of muscarinic acetylcholine receptors in the parasympathetic nervous system. Normally vagal stimulation and release of acetylcholine result in the contraction of the bronchial smooth muscle and bronchoconstriction. By blocking the muscarinic receptors, relaxation of smooth muscle occurs in the bronchi, leading to bronchodilation. The antimuscarinic drug ipratropium bromide 0.5 mg 4–6 hourly can be added to β_2-agonist therapy for patients with acute severe or life-threatening asthma or those with a poor initial response to β_2-agonist therapy (Karch 2008).

Nursing interventions

- Administer medication as prescribed and record as per policy.
- Remain with the patient giving clear explanations. Discourage lengthy conversations as the patient is short of breath.
- Fear and distress can exacerbate breathlessness and therefore the nurse should try to reassure the patient and explain the interventions required to prevent undue anxiety (Rao and Gray 2003).
- Monitor response to therapy: respiratory rate/depth/rhythm, pulse, blood pressure, O_2 saturations, work of breathing, level of consciousness, exhaustion, at least every 15 minutes or until improvement noted in patient's condition.
- Accurate recording of observations using an early warning score (EWS) is essential to assess response to treatment and highlight any deterioration in the patient's condition in a timely manner.
- Monitor peak flow readings when patient is showing a response to treatment and can perform this measurement.

- Monitor for the presence of side effects such as tachycardia, arrhythmias, tremor, hypoka-laemia and hyperglycaemia (Stanley and Tunicliffe 2008).
- Ensure prompt referral to medical staff if poor or no response to treatment observed.

Steroid therapy

Fiona was prescribed prednisolone 40 mg daily for five days orally. Corticosteroids such as prednisolone effectively reduce the airway inflammation found in virtually all patients with asthma. These drugs are equally effective when administered orally or intravenously. The oral route is preferred but may not be possible if the patient is too dyspnoeic, vomiting, or has a low level of consciousness. Corticosteroids are most effective when given within the first hour after the patient arrives in hospital and can reduce the need for hospital admission. Improvement of symptoms indicating reduction of inflammation, however, may not be seen for 2–6 hours (Pope 2011).

Nursing interventions

- Administer medication as prescribed.
- Ensure patient, and relatives if appropriate, understand the reason for administration of treatment and the need for concordance to treat the underlying inflammatory response.

Antibiotics

Fiona was prescribed antibiotics to treat an underlying chest infection which had precipitated the asthma attack.

Fluids

Fiona was also prescribed an intravenous (IV) infusion of 0.9% sodium chloride 1 litre to increase hydration and decrease the viscosity of the secretions in her airways.

Nursing interventions

- Explain the rationale for insertion of the intravenous cannula to the patient and gain consent.
- Ensure that the administration of fluids is carried out in accordance with local and national policy to prevent errors.
- Ensure cannula is securely fixed in place and maintain regular inspection of cannula insertion site to detect any signs of phlebitis.
- Record the amount of fluid administered accurately and note signs of decreasing viscosity in any sputum which patient expectorates.

5 What features should you be aware of that may indicate a life-threatening attack in a patient with severe acute asthma?

Check point: warning signs of acute asthma

- PEFR ≤33% predicted normal value or patient's personal best value
- SpO_2 <92%
- PaO_2 <8 kPa
- Normal $PaCO_2$ (4.6–6.0 kPa)
- Silent chest (absence of wheeze)
- Cyanosis
- Diminished respiratory effort
- Arrhythmia/bradycardia
- Hypotension
- Exhaustion
- Altered conscious level
- None of these features singly or together is specific and their absence does not exclude a severe attack.

(BTS and SIGN 2011)

Fiona responded to nebuliser therapy after 30 minutes and her breathlessness began to decrease; however, she was extremely tired following this acute event. She was therefore admitted for observation overnight to ensure continued response to treatment since she had demonstrated features associated with life-threatening asthma. Prior to discharge she was seen by the consultant and the asthma nurse specialist for review of medication. She was also given further education in the use of a peak flow meter and the early indications of deteriorating respiratory function. She was encouraged to visit her GP for review following discharge and seek early intervention in future to prevent further episodes of acute severe asthma.

Key points

- Patients with severe or life-threatening asthma may not always appear distressed.
- Short-acting bronchodilator drugs are the mainstay of treatment to provide relief of symptoms.
- Steroid therapy is essential to reduce inflammatory response.

REFERENCES

Aldington, S. and Beasley, R. (2007) Asthma exacerbations 5: Assessment and management of severe asthma in adults in hospital, *Thorax*, 62: 447–58.

BTS and SIGN (British Thoracic Society and Scottish Intercollegiate Guidelines Network) (2011) *British Guidelines on the Management of Asthma: Quick Reference Guide*. London: BTS.

Hunter, J. and Rawlings-Anderson, K. (2008) Respiratory assessment, *Nursing Standard*, 22(41): 41–3.

Karch, A.M. (2008) *Focus on Nursing Pharmacology*, 4th edn. Philadelphia, PA: Lippincott Williams and Wilkins.

Kennedy, S. (2007) Detecting changes in the respiratory status of ward patients, *Nursing Standard*, 21(49): 42–6.

Marotta, S.E., Belchikov, Y., Banker, K. and Marshall, P.S. (2010) Emergency management of acute severe asthma exacerbation in the adult population, *Journal of Asthma and Allergy Educators*, 1(5): 174–9.

McKenry, L., Tessier, E. and Hogan, M. (2006) *Mosby's Pharmacology in Nursing*, 22nd edn. St Louis, MO: Mosby.

Pope, B. (2011) Changing the status of acute severe asthma, *Nursing 2011 Critical Care*, 6(4): 18–25.

Porth, C.M. (2011) *Essentials of Pathophysiology: Concepts of Altered Health Status*, 3rd edn. Philadelphia, PA: Lippincott Williams and Wilkins.

Rao, A.B. and Gray, D. (2003) Breathlessness in hospitalised adult patients, *Postgraduate Medical Journal*, 79(938): 681–5.

Rees, J., Kanaber, D. and Pattani, S. (2010) *ABC of Asthma*, 6th edn. Oxford: Wiley-Blackwell BMJ Books.

Resuscitation Council (UK) (2011) *Immediate Life Support*, 3rd edn. London: Resuscitation Council (UK).

Smeltzer, S.C., Bare, B., Hinkle, J.L. and Cheever, K.H. (2008) *Brunner and Suddarth's Textbook of Medical-Surgical Nursing*, 11th edn. Philadelphia, PA: Lippincott Williams and Wilkins.

Stanley, D. and Tunicliffe, W. (2008) Management of life threatening asthma in adults: continuing education in anaesthesia, *Critical Care and Pain*, 8(3): 95–9.

Acute exacerbation of chronic obstructive pulmonary disease

Aidín McKinney

Case outline

Mary is a 69-year-old lady with a history of chronic obstructive pulmonary disease (COPD) that was diagnosed 8 years ago. Her condition is mainly characterized by a cough, with the production of some phlegm mostly in the mornings, increased shortness of breath, and she tends to fatigue easily on exertion. She has been a heavy smoker since the age of 14. She is currently on salbutamol inhalers, 2 puffs as required, and ipratropium bromide, 2 puffs four times a day. It is now winter and the weather has turned very cold in the past couple of weeks. Today she presented at her GP's surgery with symptoms of increased breathlessness, purulent sputum every time she coughs and wheezing. Her spirometry measurement was carried out and she was diagnosed with an exacerbation of her COPD. Her inhaler was changed to a long-acting beta-agonist, formoterol, to be taken twice daily and she was prescribed a seven-day course of antibiotics. She was also strongly advised to give up smoking.

---

1 **Reflect on the scenario above and define what is meant by an acute exacerbation of COPD and what could have caused this exacerbation.**

A COPD is a disease that is characterized by airflow limitation that is not fully reversible and is likely to be progressive in nature (GOLD 2011). COPD is therefore a long-term condition that has no cure, and management is largely based on the control of symptoms. The main symptoms include gradual onset of shortness of breath, particularly on exertion, along with cough and sputum production (Bostock-Cox 2010). As the condition progresses, lung function continues to decline and the underlying disease process predisposes the person to exacerbations, i.e. a temporary worsening of symptoms (Scullion and Holmes 2011). An acute exacerbation of COPD can therefore be defined as a sustained worsening of symptoms from their usual stable state which is beyond normal day-to-day variations and is acute in onset (NICE 2010). Exacerbations tend to be relatively infrequent in early COPD and therefore are mainly a feature of moderate to severe disease (Hickey 2010). Symptoms associated with an exacerbation of COPD include increased dyspnoea, increased cough, increased sputum volume and purulence, upper airway symptoms, such as colds and sore throats, increased wheeze and chest tightness, fatigue and reduced exercise tolerance. In more severe cases there may also be marked respiratory distress with possible dypsnoea, tachypnoea, cyanosis, peripheral oedema and acute confusion (NICE 2010). A higher frequency of exacerbations has been shown to correlate directly with a decline in lung function and is related to a worsening in health status and thus quality of life (Hickey 2010). This reinforces the fact that prevention and control of exacerbations are critical to the long-term management of COPD. The exact cause of an exacerbation is often unknown but generally exacerbations tend to fall into the criteria of either being the result of a viral or bacterial infection or poor air quality (Scullion and Holmes 2011). Common pathogens that are responsible are commonly *Haemophilus influenzae*, *Streptococcus pneumoniae* and *Chlamydia pneumoniae*. However, 30% or more of exacerbations are said to be attributed to the Rhinovirus or common cold, particularly in the winter months between November and March (Barnett 2007). In Mary's case, given that it is winter and that she complained of developing a cold recently, it is likely that Rhinovirus has also caused the exacerbation in this particular case. It is also likely that Mary's COPD status has progressively deteriorated and may also be attributed to the fact that she continues to smoke.

2 **Consider the initial management of Mary's condition when she visited the GP's surgery.**

A COPD is highlighted as being the most common cause of emergency hospital admissions and costs the UK economy £1.2 billion annually (Greener 2011). Early and effective management of acute exacerbations of COPD, however, is likely to prevent worsening of symptoms and promote a full recovery. Against this background, it is essential that healthcare practitioners in both community and hospital settings are aware of the revised National Institute for Health and Clinical Excellence (NICE) (2010) guidelines that highlight the recommended changes that should be made when assessing and treating patients with COPD. One of the key guidelines includes the recommendation that the treatment options should be based on the severity of the patient's condition as assessed by a combination of history taking and physical examination as well as the assessment of lung function using spirometry. Once the severity of the patient's condition is identified, NICE (2010) then recommends the treatment options that should be considered based on the most recent evidence.

In Mary's case, a history was taken; she was examined and was found to have a significant wheeze. Spirometry was also carried out. This provides an indication of airflow obstruction and is defined as a reduced forced expiratory volume in one second/forced vital capacity (FEV1/FVC) ratio (Scullion and Holmes 2010). According to NICE (2010), when carrying out spirometry, the guidelines now recommend post-bronchodilator values are measured. Mary's FEV1 was found to be >50%, post-salbutamol use and therefore in line with the revised NICE (2010) treatment algorithm for an exacerbation of COPD Mary was prescribed a long-acting beta-agonist (LABA). It was therefore recommended that she change to a formoterol inhaler twice daily and discontinue the salbutamol and ipratropium that she was currently taking. Beta-agonists work by stimulating the beta-adrenoceptors, increasing cyclic adenosine monophosphate (cAMP) concentrations, and therefore lead to relaxation of the smooth muscle to open up the airways. Long-acting beta-agonists such as formoterol are useful for exacerbations as they work for 12 hours and have an almost immediate onset of action (Bostock-Cox 2010). According to the NICE (2010) guidelines, Mary could have been prescribed a long-acting muscarinic antagonist (LAMA) instead of the formoterol, which is a long-acting beta-agonist. However, as noted by Bostock-Cox (2010), as far as choosing which long-acting bronchodilator to use, the guideline development group state that there is little difference between them based on currently available evidence, and thus which one is prescribed is mainly down to prescriber preference. The key recommendation therefore is to change from short-acting bronchodilator therapy to long-acting therapy and monitor for the response to the drug and possible adverse drug reactions. If Mary's FEV1 had been <50%, a long-acting beta-agonist drug in combination with inhaled corticosteroids should have been considered in accordance with the NICE (2010) recommendation. Thankfully, this was not warranted on this particular occasion. Mary was also prescribed a seven-day course of antibiotics. This can be useful when patients have increased breathlessness and are producing purulent sputum, as was the case with Mary. However, it is important to be aware that antibiotics should not be required if the sputum is not purulent, unless of course there are clinical signs of pneumonia or consolidation on chest X-ray (Barnett 2007).

> Later that night Mary's condition deteriorated. She was extremely short of breath, and found it difficult to even get herself ready for bed. She was visited by the out-of-hours doctor who noted that she was using pursed lip breathing and her accessory muscles in an effort to improve her breathing and consequently arranged for her to be admitted to hospital. On admission to hospital, she was very short of breath, and her oxygen saturation level was 86% on room air.

3 **Discuss how you would assess Mary's breathing and the severity of this particular exacerbation.**

A An assessment of the severity of Mary's breathing and indeed the severity of this exacerbation of her COPD should be based on Mary's medical history before the exacerbation, as well as focusing on the symptoms themselves.

- *History*: It is important to consider for how long the new symptoms have been present, what exactly these are compared to Mary's previous symptoms, and whether they are causing any limitation to daily activities. It would also be useful to ascertain whether there had been any previous episodes of exacerbations and whether or not hospitalization was required as a result of these. A history of past and present treatment regimes would also be useful (Britton 2002).
- *Signs and symptoms*: According to NICE (2010), signs of a severe exacerbation of COPD may include marked dyspnoea, tachypnoea, pursed lip breathing, use of accessory muscles, acute confusion, and marked reduction in activities of daily living, some of which were apparent in Mary's case. It was therefore evident that in view of these symptoms, a hospital admission was warranted. An ABCDE assessment should also be undertaken given the acute nature of Mary's condition. Assessment of Mary's airway and breathing should in particular consider the presence of wheeze, the presence of a cough, the production of sputum and the degree of breathlessness as well as obtaining values such as the respiratory rate, spirometry values, oxygen saturation levels and an arterial blood gas. Some of these will be considered in more detail below.
- *Measurement of breathlessness*: Various tools are available that measure the degree of breathlessness; however, the Medical Research Council (MRC) dyspnoea scale is

considered to be particularly useful as it focuses on assessing the degree of breathlessness experienced by the patient themselves (Bostock-Cox 2010). The MRC dyspnoea scale therefore allows patients to grade their breathlessness on a scale of 1–5 according to the activity carried out. Thus, Grade 1 refers to 'not troubled by breathlessness except on strenuous exercise' and Grade 5 indicates 'too breathless to leave the house, or breathless when dressing or undressing'. It is therefore an easy-to-use tool that allows the practitioner to ascertain a baseline assessment of the current degree of breathlessness as well as monitoring for any improvement or deterioration (Barnett 2007). Given that Mary was experiencing breathlessness that was impinging on her ability to carry out normal activities of daily living such as getting ready for bed, it is apparent that her degree of breathlessness was at Grade 5.

- *Oxygen saturations*: Oxygen saturation levels are also important to consider. Patients are likely to experience low oxygen saturation levels at rest and/or on exertion as their COPD progresses. If oxygen saturation levels are <93%, as was the case with Mary, an arterial blood gas should be taken and oxygen therapy considered (Barnett 2007). Administration of oxygen therapy in the case of COPD will be considered in more detail below.

- *Activities of daily living*: Severity of the patient's breathlessness will obviously determine the ability to carry out daily tasks. As already noted, Mary was having difficulty getting ready for bed and consequently it is likely that the breathlessness will also impact on many other activities of daily living. It is therefore useful to carry out a baseline assessment using nursing models of care, such as the Roper, Logan and Tierney model to establish the impact on daily activities both now and prior to the exacerbation (Elsherif and Noble 2011). However, given that Mary is currently experiencing severe shortness of breath, the assessment will need to be limited to using closed yes/no questions and a fuller assessment will have to wait until this acute episode is relieved.

- *Level of responsiveness*: In a patient with a severe exacerbation of their COPD, it is also important to closely monitor the patient's alertness and level of responsiveness. Any deterioration in this, including increased drowsiness and/or confusion, may be indicative of increased levels of hypoxia (Britton 2002).

4   **Discuss the administration of oxygen therapy to Mary given that she has COPD.**

A   Mary is obviously in acute respiratory distress, therefore the main aim is to enable Mary to breathe comfortably again and maintain her oxygen saturation levels above 90%. As recommended by NICE (2010), if the oxygen saturation level is below 92% in a patient with COPD, oxygen therapy should always be considered. However, it is imperative to remember that oxygen therapy should always be used with caution with COPD patients as in some COPD patients their respiratory drive depends on their degree of hypoxia rather than the usual dependence on hypercapnia. In such patients, it is therefore important to be aware that uncontrolled oxygen therapy can result in suppression of the respiratory drive and lead to the patient developing a respiratory arrest. For this reason, it is best to proceed cautiously and start off by administering 28% oxygen (via a venturi mask/4 litres per minute) in a patient with COPD until their arterial blood gas is checked. However, if the patient is showing signs of hypoxia, the healthcare professional may need to quickly proceed to giving high flow oxygen. If this is the case, it is vital that the arterial blood gases (ABGs) are promptly checked (NICE 2010). It is useful to point out that patients whose respiratory drive depends on their degree of hypoxia are rarely encountered in practice but the possibility of this occurring in patients with severe COPD should always be considered. However, by the same token, the consequences of severe hypoxia in COPD patients is also not fully appreciated and has resulted in inadequate oxygen therapy being administered to a number of COPD patients and in some cases this has resulted in death from hypoxia occurring (NICE 2010).

Thus, in Mary's case, it would be advisable to maintain Mary in as upright a position as possible and start off by administering oxygen at 28% (via a venturi mask/4 litres per minute) and progressively increasing it until her oxygen saturations reach 85–90% or her pO$_2$ increases to within normal levels as checked on the arterial blood gas. If, however, the oxygen saturation levels continue to remain below 85% or she shows signs of hypoxia, e.g. cyanosis, it may then become necessary to administer high flow oxygen at 15 litres per minute via a non-rebreathing mask. Full observations of her vital signs should also be recorded every 15 minutes. This must include observation of her oxygen saturation levels and her respiratory effort to ensure that the oxygen therapy is showing signs of effectiveness, that the oxygen saturation levels are rising above 85% or reaching the target range for the particular patient and the patient is not developing further hypoxia. After giving oxygen for 30–60 minutes, the arterial blood gas should be rechecked to allow for the detection of any further increase in carbon dioxide concentrations or falling pH levels. If this occurs, or Mary's breathing or oxygen saturation levels deteriorate further, it is imperative that the medical team is contacted again and the patient assessed promptly and consideration given to further intervention such as nebuliser therapy and/or transfer to high dependency or intensive care (Elsherif and Noble 2011).

After four days in hospital, Mary's condition was much improved and she was to be discharged home.

5   **What discharge advice and follow-up care are required to help prevent Mary from developing further exacerbations?**

A   The NICE guidelines suggest that the frequency and indeed the impact of exacerbations could perhaps be reduced by giving better self-management advice to patients and providing encouragement to develop the skills needed to recognize the early symptoms of an exacerbation and know how to respond appropriately (Booker 2004). In view of this, it is recommended that pulmonary rehabilitation be made available to all patients who consider themselves disabled by their lung function (NICE 2004). New to the 2010 guidelines was also the proviso that pulmonary rehabilitation be made available to all appropriate people with COPD, including those who have had a recent hospitalization for an acute exacerbation, as was the case with Mary (NICE 2010). Pulmonary rehabilitation should take the form of an organized multidisciplinary programme of care that takes place over a period of six to eight weeks and should incorporate advice on exercise, disease education, vaccination advice, nutrition and psychological and behavioural intervention, including smoking cessation (Booker 2004; Scullion and Holmes 2010). Some of these points will be discussed further below.

SMOKING CESSATION

Smoking cessation is identified as being one of the most important elements in the management of COPD and stopping smoking should significantly reduce exacerbations. All COPD patients, regardless of their age, should therefore be encouraged to stop smoking and given help to do so. This may include encouraging patients to attend smoking cessation groups, offering nicotine replacement therapy, or varenicline or bupropion (unless contraindicated) combined with a support programme at every available opportunity (Scullion and Holmes 2010). As Mary is a heavy smoker, it is essential that smoking cessation is encouraged to reduce her risk of further and possibly more severe exacerbations in the future.

VACCINATION

Influenza or pneumococcal vaccination may also be useful in order to help prevent an exacerbation, particularly in the winter months. If Mary had availed herself of such a vaccination, she might have avoided this particular infective episode.

EDUCATION

Patients should be provided with relevant information and including education on the risk factors for exacerbations of COPD, such as continuing to smoke, developing a respiratory infection, declining FEV1 levels, falling body mass index, number of previous hospitalizations for COPD and long-term oxygen therapy. Patients should also be advised on how to recognize an exacerbation and what to do if an exacerbation occurs, including an awareness of some of the key measures that may be employed to effectively manage an exacerbation, such as prompt increase in bronchodilator therapy and possible use of antibiotics and steroids (Scullion and Holmes 2011). In a study by Kessler et al. (2006), it was noted that exacerbations vary greatly between patients; however, the symptoms are generally consistent in individuals and the majority of patients can recognize the warning signs. In view of this, it seems to suggest that self-management plans and education could be useful to promote earlier intervention and reduce exacerbations.

EXERCISE/SOCIAL INTERACTION

It is also recommended that all patients with COPD should be encouraged to take regular exercise such as walking, assisted if necessary. Patients may require encouragement to consider what they are capable of doing, rather than focusing on what they cannot do. Otherwise many are likely to enter a downward spiral of breathlessness, inactivity, social isolation and apathy (Britton 2002). Exercise is also important from a nutritional perspective as it helps to improve the patient's appetite and stimulates the anabolic response required to increase lean body mass. NICE (2010) therefore suggests that individuals with COPD should be encouraged to take physical exercise in order to augment the effects of nutrition.

NUTRITION

Weight loss, in particular, loss of fat-free mass, is common in patients with COPD, especially as the disease progresses. If left untreated, this can lead to cachexia, which is characterized by substantial weight loss and muscle wasting. Factors that may contribute to weight loss in COPD patients include possible dysphagia and problems with chewing due to dyspnoea, excess mucus production, coughing spasms leading to retching and vomiting, and lack of motivation/effort in food preparation when already lethargic (Shepherd 2010). Obesity also poses difficulties for the COPD patient. Kelly (2007) suggests that an excess of intra-abdominal fat can prevent full expansion of the lungs, leading to dyspnoea and further discomfort in individuals with existing COPD. Assessment of nutritional status and promotion of optimal nutrition should therefore be an important element in the management of COPD. It is essential that diet and also the importance of exercise are therefore discussed with all COPD patients such as Mary prior to discharge (Shepherd 2010).

Key points

- Main causes of acute exacerbations of COPD result from either viral or bacterial infection.
- Early and effective management of acute exacerbations are likely to prevent worsening of symptoms and promote a full recovery.
- Oxygen should always be administered cautiously in COPD patients; however, at times high levels of oxygen therapy may be required to prevent hypoxia.

REFERENCES

Barnett, M. (2007) An overview of assessment and management in COPD, *British Journal of Community Nursing*, 14(5): 195–201.

Booker, R. (2004) New guidelines for the management of COPD, *Practice Nursing*, 15(3): 130–4.

Bostock-Cox, B. (2010) Prescribing inhaled therapies in the treatment of COPD, *Nurse Prescribing*, 8(12): 571–7.

Britton, M. (2002) Preventing and treating acute episodes of COPD, *Practice Nursing*, 13(11): 482–9.

Elsherif, M. and Noble, H. (2011) Management of COPD using the Roper-Logan-Tierney framework, *British Journal of Nursing*, 20(1): 29–33.

GOLD (Global Initiative for Chronic Obstructive Lung Disease) (2011) *Global Strategy for the Diagnosis, Management and Prevention of Chronic Obstructive Pulmonary Disease*. Available at: www.goldcopd.com (accessed 17 January 2012).

Greener, M. (2011) Easing the burden of COPD: NICE guidelines and new agents, *Nurse Prescribing*, 2: 64–7.

Hickey, S. (2010) Strategies for reducing exacerbations of COPD, *Practice Nursing*, 21(2): 78–83.

Kelly, C. (2007) Optimising nutrition in COPD, *British Journal of Primary Care Nursing*, 1(3): 117–20. Available at: www.bjpcn-respiratory.com/download/2713.

Kessler, R., Stahl, E., Vogelmeier, C., Haughney, J., Trudeau, E., Lofdahl, C. and Partridge, M.R. (2006) Patient understanding, detection and experience of COPD, *Chest*, 130(1): 133–42.

NICE (National Institute for Health and Clinical Excellence) (2004) *Quick Reference Guide: Chronic Obstructive Pulmonary Disease: Management of Chronic Obstructive Pulmonary Disease in Adults in Primary and Secondary Care*, Clinical Guideline 12. London: NICE.

NICE (National Institute for Health and Clinical Excellence) (2010) *Chronic Obstructive Pulmonary Disease: Management of Chronic Obstructive Pulmonary Disease in Adults in Primary and Secondary Care*. Available at: http://Rguidance.nice.org.uk (accessed 7 June 2011).

Scullion, J. and Holmes, S. (2010) Chronic obstructive pulmonary disease (COPD): updated guidelines, *Primary Healthcare*, 20(8): 33–40.

Scullion, J. and Holmes, S. (2011) Strategies to reduce COPD exacerbations, *Practice Nursing*, 22(2): 83–6.

Shepherd, A. (2010) The nutritional management of COPD: an overview, *British Journal of Nursing*, 19(9): 559–62.

Pulmonary embolism
Karen Page

Case outline

Alison Cairns, a 72-year-old lady, was receiving treatment from the district nurse for varicose ulcers on her left and right legs. She had a history of type 2 diabetes and hypertension and was moderately overweight. The district nurse was currently visiting her twice weekly to re-dress the ulcers which were causing her quite a lot of pain and discomfort. This was restricting her ability to go out and about although she was managing to walk around the house with the help of a walking aid independently. Her niece visited Alison usually every other day to bring groceries and leave ready prepared meals for her aunt. On her latest visit to see Alison, the district nurse became concerned that the patient's general condition had deteriorated and she considered that her leg ulcers required more intensive treatment. She also felt that her right leg in particular was showing signs of developing marked cellulitis. She contacted the GP who felt that it was appropriate to refer Alison to the local hospital and so she was admitted directly to the medical ward later that evening for further assessment of her condition.

You are working on the ward that evening and when you meet Alison, she states that she really doesn't feel very well today and that she was finding it increasingly difficult to cope at home due to the deterioration in the condition of her legs. Alison appears anxious and you note that she seems to be short of breath on minimal exertion. There was no evidence of wheeze associated with this although she did acknowledge some chest discomfort associated with respiration which she indicates is unusual for her.

---

1 **What is your initial course of action?**

A As this patient is a direct admission to the ward, it is essential to consider the fact that she should be properly assessed in order to establish the full extent of the patient's problems. An initial ABCDE assessment will reveal any urgent problems which require immediate management. Reassurance should also be provided to address any anxiety surrounding her admission to hospital and her dyspnoea. The nurse should also remember to confirm with her that her next of kin, in this case her niece, has been informed of her admission. As this is an elderly lady who lives alone and has restricted mobility, the nurse must also be aware of the holistic nature of the assessment which must be carried out once the patient's condition has been stabilized, to establish any other potential physical or social problems which will require attention in preparation for discharge. However, in view of the fact that she is short of breath and states that she does not feel very well at present, this should be postponed until her preliminary problems have been dealt with. It is important that the medical staff are made aware of her admission and that your clinical findings are reported immediately using a recognized communication tool such as SBAR. The patient should also be commenced on an early warning score (EWS) chart to facilitate ongoing monitoring of her condition.

Following an assessment, the following clinical observations are recorded. Alison is alert and orientated but appears very anxious and agitated. Her clinical observations are:

Temperature: 37.4°C
Pulse: 110 beats per minute
Respiration rate: 24 breaths per minute
Oxygen saturations: 93% on room air
Blood pressure: 140/86mmHg.

An ECG was also recorded. Oxygen was administered as prescribed to maintain saturations of >96% and the patient positioned to aid chest expansion.

On inspection, the right leg appears swollen and the patient reports that although the ulcers had been healing, the right leg ulcer in particular has broken down again over the last week and has become very painful which has restricted her mobility significantly over the past few days. You notice that her left leg is also swollen (left calf measured 3 cm more than the right calf) and appears to be quite red and warm to touch. Alison states that this is also a recent occurrence as this ulcer was smaller than the other and seemed to be healing well.

2   **What information can be obtained from this initial clinical assessment that may point to possible causes of the onset of Alison's shortness of breath and chest discomfort?**

A   The ECG should be reviewed urgently since the patient is complaining of some chest discomfort. Chest discomfort can be associated with cardiopulmonary or other problems which require immediate attention, e.g. acute coronary syndrome and respiratory problems. Chest discomfort may even be due to musculoskeletal pain or gastric causes such as reflux which must also be eliminated from the list of possible diagnoses. Alison's ECG did not demonstrate any evidence of acute coronary syndrome; however, the ECG confirmed the presence of sinus tachycardia. It was therefore essential to seek other explanations of the patient's chest discomfort. Abnormalities including tachycardia and nonspecific ST and T wave abnormalities can be seen in pulmonary embolism (PE) though it is acknowledged that the ECG is a poor diagnostic tool for PE; however, anterior T wave inversion is thought to have a sensitivity of approximately 85% in cases of pulmonary embolism (Farley et al. 2009). Moreover, in addition to her chest symptoms Alison demonstrated some indication of the possibility of having a deep venous thrombosis (DVT) on initial clinical examination. More than 90% of pulmonary emboli are the consequence of clots that were formed in the deep veins of the legs and pelvis. Calf asymmetry of more than 1 cm increases the likelihood of a deep venous thrombosis from 27% to 56% in at-risk individuals (McCance and Huether 2006). Alison's left leg was noticeably swollen on admission with a difference of 3 cm in the measurement of the right and left calf and she was complaining of some pain in this leg, which suggested the presence of a DVT. It is important to remember, however, that although characteristic symptoms of DVT are leg pain and swelling, DVT is often asymptomatic and the findings may be subtle. British Thoracic Society guidelines (BTS 2003) suggest that if the patient has clinical features compatible with a PE such as breathlessness and tachypnoea with the presence of a major risk factor for venous thromboembolism such as a DVT, the probability of a pulmonary embolism being present is high. This is extremely significant and must be taken very seriously because, if left untreated, the patient has the potential to become acutely ill and deteriorate very quickly due to a further embolic event. Further investigations were therefore required to confirm the presence of a potential PE in Alison's case to facilitate ongoing care.

3   **Discuss the most common tests used to assist in the diagnosis of pulmonary embolism.**

A   The most common tests used are as follows:

- *D-dimer*: As a thrombus or embolism begins to break down, fibrin degradation products are released into the blood stream. One of these products is D-dimer. Normally plasma contains no detectable amount of D-dimer and therefore if it is present, it indicates clot breakdown (Farley et al. 2009). A positive diagnosis of DVT or PE cannot be made on the basis of D-dimer alone, however, as levels can be raised in other conditions such as during infection, malignancy, pregnancy and following surgery (Welch 2006). Nevertheless, a positive result does indicate the need for further investigation.
- *Chest X-ray*: A chest X-ray is often normal in cases of pulmonary embolism; however, it can be used to rule out other pathology.
- *Leg ultrasound*: Since 70% of patients with proven PE have proximal DVT, leg ultrasound has been used in suspected PE as an initial test in those with the presence of clinical signs and symptoms of DVT. Duplex ultrasonography is a non-invasive investigation which can demonstrate the speed of blood flow through the veins and reveal evidence of clot formation. It also allows indirect visualization of the structure of the patient's leg veins. A Doppler ultrasound of Alison's left leg revealed a deep venous thrombosis in the popliteal vein.
- *Ventilation/perfusion scan (V/Q scan)*: This nuclear medicine test is used to demonstrate under-perfused areas of the lung. The patient inhales radioactive gas and receives an injection of radioactive material. By following these substances through the lungs and the remainder of the body, it is possible to demonstrate areas of the lung with less uptake of the material which alters the relationship between ventilation and perfusion of the lung tissue known as the V/Q ratio (Shaughnessy 2007). A normal scan reliably excludes PE; however, it must be remembered that although a high probability result usually indicates a PE, a significant minority of high probability results are false positives. Therefore, it is important that any result is taken in conjunction with the clinical picture of the patient (BTS 2003). In many places this test has now been replaced by CT scanning.
- *Computed tomographic pulmonary angiography (CTPA)*: CTPA is now widely available and can be used to determine the exact location and measurements of a PE. It is now the recommended initial lung imaging modality for non-massive PE if the patient's condition permits (Farley et al. 2009).

4 **Discuss the origins of a pulmonary embolism and identify the three factors which are thought to contribute to an increased risk of development of this condition. Consider how these are demonstrated in Alison's case.**

A In normal circumstances, microthrombi which form in the venous system are constantly broken down through natural fibrinolytic processes. These processes ensure that local haemostasis is maintained and prevent uninhibited clotting. DVT and PE are often referred to as venous thromboembolism. Almost all pulmonary emboli arise from deep vein thrombosis in the large veins of the lower legs, typically originating in the popliteal vein or larger veins above it (Porth 2011). Throughout the venous system, vessels converge rather than branch as blood flows into increasingly larger vessels until it returns to the heart. Emboli that are carried in the systemic venous return therefore have little possibility of occluding a vessel on the way back to the heart. However, from the right side of the heart they are pumped into the pulmonary arterial system. As these vessels branch, the emboli ultimately come to a smaller artery which they cannot pass through. PE develops when a blood-borne substance, usually a thrombus or part of a thrombus (embolus), lodges in a branch of the pulmonary artery and obstructs blood flow (Porth 2011).

Three factors are considered to contribute to thrombosis formation: (1) venous stasis; (2) hypercoagulability; and (3) injury to the vascular endothelium. These are collectively known as Virchow's triad (Farley et al. 2009):

1 *Venous stasis*: Peripheral veins and especially the leg veins rely on the skeletal muscles to assist blood flow. As muscles contract, they shorten and thicken, compressing the veins that pass over and between them. In conjunction with the veins' internal system of valves, this makes a major contribution to venous return from the legs. Venous stasis is usually caused by immobility associated with prolonged bed rest or sitting, obesity, neurological disease or old age. Reduction or lack of normal physical activity slows the rate of circulation because of decreased demand by the muscles and more importantly because of the loss of skeletal muscle pumping. Blood hyperviscosity and heart conditions such as heart failure may also contribute to venous stasis (Farley et al. 2009).

2 *Hypercoagulability*: This can result from inherited, or acquired coagulation, disorders of the blood, pregnancy, malignancy or contraceptive use. However, in some cases, the reasons underpinning this disorder remain obscure (McCance and Huether 2006).

3 *Endothelial damage or injury*: Damage to the vessel wall can be caused by trauma, bone fractures and dislocations, chemical injury with sclerosing agents, contrast agents or intravenous injections. The presence of central venous catheters, previous deep venous thrombosis or PE, and toxins such as those released in sepsis can also contribute to endothelial damage (Race and Collier 2007).

> Alison clearly had a number of risk factors for PE as she was over 70 years of age and had become increasingly immobile due to the recent deterioration in her leg ulcers. She was also demonstrating indications of the presence of deep vein thrombosis in her lower left leg.

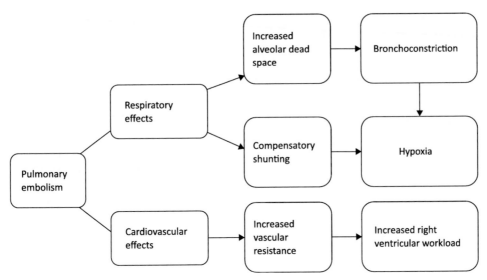

Figure 5.1 Effects of blockage of the pulmonary arterial system

5 **Discuss the potential pathological effects of a pulmonary embolism.**

A The pathological effects of pulmonary thromboembolism depend largely on the size of the embolism and degree of pulmonary blood flow obstruction (Porth 2011). Pulmonary embolism can be classified as small/medium pulmonary embolism, massive or recurrent. In the small/medium embolism, the embolism has impacted in a terminal pulmonary vessel which should be survivable. In a massive P E, sudden collapse will occur. The largest clots can result in sudden death by obstructing right ventricular outflow (Race and Collier 2007). In recurrent P E, there is often increased breathlessness occurring over weeks (Kumar and Clarke 2005).

Blockage of the pulmonary arterial system has both pulmonary and haemodynamic consequences (Figure 5.1). The effects on the pulmonary system are increased alveolar dead space, bronchoconstriction, and compensatory shunting. The haemodynamic effects include an increase in pulmonary vascular resistance and right ventricular workload (Urden et al. 2008).

RESPIRATORY EFFECTS

Increased dead space

An increase in alveolar dead space occurs because an area of the lung is being ventilated but not perfused. This leads to an increase in the work of breathing. To limit the amount of alveolar dead space, localized bronchoconstriction occurs.

Compensatory shunting

Compensatory shunting occurs because the unaffected areas of the lungs have to accommodate the entire cardiac output. This creates a situation in which perfusion exceeds ventilation and blood is returned to the left side of the heart without participating in gas exchange which leads to the development of hypoxaemia (Urden et al. 2008).

HAEMODYNAMIC CONSEQUENCES

Increased pulmonary vascular resistance

The major haemodynamic consequence of a PE is the development of pulmonary hypertension which is partly related to the actual mechanical obstruction of the pulmonary vascular bed itself. The development of hypoxia causes pulmonary vasoconstriction which further exacerbates pulmonary hypertension. As pulmonary hypertension increases, so does the work of the right ventricle which is reflected by a rise in pulmonary artery pressure. Consequently right ventricular failure occurs which can lead to a decrease in left ventricular preload, a decrease in blood pressure and, in the case of a massive embolism, the development of shock and subsequent death (Urden et al. 2008).

A CTPA revealed evidence of a pulmonary embolism and Alison was therefore commenced on treatment. She was prescribed a low molecular weight heparin (LMWH) initially and subsequently prescribed the oral anticoagulant drug warfarin.

---

6 **Discuss the function of anticoagulant therapy in the treatment of PE and identify how this is monitored.**

A If a massive thrombus has formed in the pulmonary circulation, it is essential to dissolve the clot without delay to restore blood flow to the affected tissues. In this case, thrombolytic agents may be prescribed. However, in less severe cases which nevertheless require urgent treatment to prevent further or potentially more serious events, anticoagulant drugs will be prescribed. These drugs do not prevent platelet plug formation nor do they break down clots that have already formed. Anticoagulant drugs, however, interfere with the normal coagulation process to slow or prevent further clot formation, thus assisting in the prevention of further thromboembolic episodes. The two main groups of anticoagulant drugs are: (1) parenteral anticoagulant drugs; and (2) oral anticoagulant drugs.

The parenteral anticoagulant drugs include heparin and the low molecular weight heparins. Heparin is a naturally occurring substance that inhibits the conversion of prothrombin to thrombin, thus blocking the conversion of fibrinogen to fibrin which is the final step in clot formation. It is given via the intravenous route and has an almost immediate onset of action. The low molecular weight heparins are isolated from standard heparin and have more specific antithrombin activity by activating antifactor Xa (McKenry et al. 2006). They have a longer duration of action allowing them to be prescribed once or twice daily via subcutaneous injection. This means that they do not usually require routine monitoring.

Heparin is monitored by using either partial prothrombin time (PTT) or activated partial prothrombin time (aPPT). The aPPT is a more sensitive version of the PTT and is more commonly used. The aPPT is used to identify deficiencies in the intrinsic coagulation system and evaluate the efficacy of heparin therapy. The goal is to have aPPT 1.5–2.5 times the normal laboratory control value to ensure the effectiveness of the drug.

Subsequently patients will be placed on long-term protective anticoagulant therapy within 24 hours of initial treatment (Farley et al. 2009). The oral anticoagulant most commonly used is warfarin. Warfarin interferes with the production of vitamin K-dependent clotting factors which are required in the clotting cascade. Warfarin is monitored using prothrombin time/international normalized ratio (INR). Prothrombin is a vitamin K-dependent protein produced by the liver and involved in coagulation. The target range for prevention of most thromboembolic events is 2.5 (range 2–3). The INR result reflects a warfarin dose adminis-tered 36–72 hours prior to testing (McKenry et al. 2006). In view of this time delay, it must be stressed that warfarin is not the drug of choice in the acute situation but is used to main-tain long-term anticoagulation therapy.

7 **Identify the patient safety issues which should be the focus of the nursing management associated with the administration of anticoagulant therapy. Provide a rationale for your answer.**

A Table 5.1 shows the rationale behind the nursing management decisions in anticoagulant therapy.

Table 5.1 Rationale for nursing management decisions in anticoagulant therapy

Nursing management	Rationale
Prior to administration of anticoagulant therapy, review the patient's medication for the presence of allergies or significant drug interactions	Increased bleeding can occur if heparin is combined with drugs such as oral anticoagulants or NSAIDS. Decreased anticoagulation can occur if heparin is combined with glyceryl trinitrate (GTN) (BNF 2011). Warfarin has a significant number of interactions with other drugs. It is therefore important to recognize that drugs should not be added or taken away from a patient's drug regime without careful monitoring or adjustment of the dosage to prevent serious adverse effects. It is important to consult a current *British National Formulary* (BNF) for further guidelines and information
Identify any pre-existing conditions such as GI ulcers, haemorrhagic disorders or recent surgery	These conditions may be exacerbated by increased clotting times leading to a risk of bleeding
Ensure laboratory tests such as a full blood picture including haematocrit and platelets are performed before initiation of therapy	To establish a baseline prior to therapy and ensure that any adverse effects can be quickly evaluated and detected. Heparin can lead to thrombocytopenia so it is vital to monitor platelet levels during therapy (BNF 2011)
Regularly monitor vital signs including BP, pulse and respiratory rate	A drop in blood pressure or haematocrit levels can also indicate bleeding (Palatnik 2007)

(Continued overleaf)

Table 5.1 (*Continued*)

Nursing management	Rationale
Regularly monitor urea and electrolytes, liver function tests, renal function tests	Reduced liver and renal function can lead to the need for reduced or altered dosage
The patient's gums, skin, urine and faeces should be observed for signs of overt or occult bleeding. Signs of nosebleeds, petechiae or bruising should also be reported promptly to the prescriber	These signs may indicate the drug dosage is incorrect and requires review
Monitor the patient's INR or aPTT laboratory values	To ensure that the drug levels remain within the therapeutic range
Provide safety precautions against bleeding such as the use of an electric razor. Keep venepuncture and injection sites to a minimum	The state of increased anticoagulation increases the risk of blood loss and bruising
Ensure that the antidotes to both heparin and warfarin are readily available	Protamine sulphate is the antidote to heparin and vitamin K is the antidote to warfarin (McKenry et al. 2006). These should be available in the case of an overdose of the drug which has the potential to lead to severe haemorrhage
Provide patient education	To enhance the patient's knowledge and understanding about the purpose of the drug therapy and to promote concordance with the drug regime
Discuss the need to inform not only their own GP but also their pharmacist and dentist to the fact that they are receiving anticoagulant therapy. Discuss the advisability of wearing MedicAlert bracelets	To alert health care personnel to the fact that the patient is receiving anticoagulant therapy and the need for vigilance with respect to drug interactions or prolonged bleeding times

Alison was successfully treated with a low molecular weight heparin and commenced on long-term warfarin therapy which will be monitored by the district nurse and her G P. She was reviewed by the tissue viability nurse specialist to provide advice on enhancing wound healing. Following a period of intensive treatment the ulcers were sufficiently improved to reduce the pain she was experiencing, thus also enhancing her mobility prior to discharge.

Key points

- Pulmonary embolism has the potential to cause fatality if the embolism blocks a major pulmonary artery.
- Many patients with P E will demonstrate evidence of DVT.
- Anticoagulant therapy is required to prevent further episodes of P E.

REFERENCES

BNF (British National Formulary) (2011) *BNF 62*, September. London: BMJ Group and Pharmaceutical Press.

British Thoracic Society Standards of Care Committee Pulmonary Embolism Guideline Development Group (2003) British Thoracic Society guidelines for the management of suspected acute pulmonary embolism, *Thorax*, 58: 470–84.

Farley, A.H. et al. (2009) Pulmonary embolism: identification, clinical features and management, *Nursing Standard*, 23(28): 49–56.

Kumar, P. and Clark, M. (2005) *Clinical Medicine*, 6th edn. London: Elsevier Saunders.

McCance, K.L. and Huether, S.E. (2006) *Pathophysiology: The Biologic Basis for Disease in Adults and Children*, 5th edn. St Louis, MO: Elsevier Mosby.

McKenry, L., Tessier, E. and Hogan, M. (2006) *Mosby's Pharmacology in Nursing*, 22nd edn. St Louis, MO: Mosby.

Palatnik, A. (2007) Putting a stop to thrombi, *Nursing*, 37(Suppl. Cardiac): 2–6.

Porth, C.M. (2011) *Essentials of Pathophysiology*, 3rd edn. Philadelphia, PA: Lippincott Williams and Wilkins.

Race, T.K. and Collier, P.E. (2007) The hidden risk of deep vein thrombosis: the need for risk factor assessment, *Critical Care Nursing Quarterly*, 30(3): 245–54.

Shaughnessy, K. (2007) Massive pulmonary embolism, *Critical Care Nurse*, 27: 39–50.

Urden, L.D., Stacy, K.M. and Lough, M.E. (2008) *Priorities in Critical Care Nursing*, 5th edn. St Louis, MO: Mosby Elsevier.

Welch, E. (2006) The assessment and management of venous thromboembolism, *Nursing Standard*, 20(28): 58–64.

PART 3
Renal System

Acute kidney injury
Aidín McKinney

Case outline

John Brown is a 72-year-old man (100 kg) who has recently returned to the general surgical ward following a resection of part of his bowel. His past medical history includes smoking for 40 years (but not in the past 10 years), hypertension, and diabetes (type 2) that was diagnosed 5 years ago. His current medication includes ramipril 2.5 mg and gliclazide 40 mg twice daily. He also reports that he takes non-steroidal anti-inflammatory drugs (NSAIDs) regularly due to chronic back pain. Overall the surgery was uneventful although it was estimated that he sustained a 2-litre blood loss. He was transfused with 2 units of blood alongside other intravenous fluids. On return to the ward his condition appeared stable. He has two redivac drains in situ and there was minimal drainage noted in them. His vital signs were also within normal limits. Later that afternoon, however, the nursing staff noted that his urinary output had decreased to less than 40 mL/hour. They continued to monitor this for a couple of hours and then informed the doctor when it showed no signs of improvement. Bloods were sent off to the laboratory as the doctor was concerned that John might be developing acute kidney injury (AKI). The results are highlighted below.

Biochemistry:
Sodium: 137 mmol/L (135–145 mmol/L)
Potassium: 4.5 mmol/L (3.4–5.1 mmol/L)
Urea: 7.6 mmol/L (1.7–8.3 mmol/L)
Creatinine: 98 μmol/L (female 50–90 μmol/L, male 70–120 μmol/L)
Calcium: 2.6 mmol/L (2.2–2.5 mmol/L).

---

1   **Reflect on the scenario above and consider whether or not John may be diagnosed as having now developed acute kidney injury.**

A   The term acute kidney injury (AKI) replaces what was previously described and indeed is still often referred to as acute renal failure (ARF) (Davenport et al. 2008). This shift in terminology was driven mainly by the need to emphasize the importance of less severe impairment of kidney function and the benefits of early detection rather than focusing on the kidney's inability to perform glomerular filtration as the term ARF suggests (Davies 2009). Furthermore, it was argued that too many different definitions of acute renal failure existed in the literature. In view of this, the Acute Dialysis Quality Initiative (ADQI), a group of international specialists in nephrology and intensive care, developed a definition and classification system for AKI in 2004 known as the RIFLE criteria (see Table 6.1). This classification system outlines three levels of severity: risk, injury and failure; and two outcomes: loss and end-stage kidney disease (ESKD). It therefore challenges the perception that renal dysfunction is not only regarded as being important when it reaches the point of failure but rather is a spectrum that varies from risk to end-stage kidney disease (Murphy and Byrne 2010). The Acute Kidney Injury Network (AKIN), another group of experts, refined these RIFLE criteria and renamed the stages as one, two and three, with stage three categorizing any patient requiring renal replacement therapy (see Table 6.2). The UK Renal Association has adopted the AKIN criteria and definition of AKI. AKI is defined by AKIN as an abrupt reduction in kidney function as identified by any one of the following:

- Serum creatinine rising ≥26.4 micromol/litre within 48 hours.
- A rise in serum creatinine ≥150–200% (1.5–2 fold) within 48 hours.
- Urine output <0.5 mL/kg/hour for more than 6 hours (Davenport et al. 2008).

It is interesting to note that urea is noticeably not included in this definition. Urea, together with serum creatinine and urinary output, were traditionally viewed as the preferred markers for assessing ARF; however, it is now recognized that urea levels may be raised for non-renal reasons and therefore are not included in the definition (Woodrow 2009). Creatinine, a waste product of muscle metabolism (hence gender differences in normal value levels), however, remains a useful marker. Creatinine is normally cleared in urine, therefore, in kidney injury levels usually rise steadily by 50–100 micromoles for each day of failure. However, it is also important to be aware that blood creatinine varies throughout

Table 6.1 The RIFLE classification for AKI

Class	Glomerular filtration rate (GFR) criteria	Urinary output criteria
R = Risk	Increased serum creatinine × 1.5 baseline Or GFR decreases ≥25%	<0.5 mL/kg/hr for 6 hours
I = Injury	Increased serum creatinine × 2 baseline Or GFR decreases ≥50%	<0.5 mL/kg/hr for 12 hours
F = Failure	Increased serum creatinine × 3 baseline Or GFR decreases ≥75% Or serum creatinine ≥354 µmol/L with an acute rise of at least 44 µmol/L	<0.3 mL/kg/hr for 24 hours Or anuria for 12 hours
L = Loss	Persistent acute renal failure = complete loss of kidney function >4 weeks	
E = ESKD	End-stage kidney disease >3 months	

Source: Bellomo et al. (2004); Murphy and Byrne (2010).

Table 6.2 The Acute Kidney Injury Network diagnostic criteria for AKI

AKIN stage	Serum creatinine (SCr) criteria	Urine output criteria
1	Increase in SCr ≥26.4 µmol/L Or Increase in SCr ≥150–200% (1.5–2 fold) from baseline	<0.5 mL/kg/hr for 6 hours
2	Increase in SCr >200–300% (>2–3 fold) from baseline	<0.5 mL/kg/hr for 12 hours
3	Increase in SCr >300% (>3 fold) from baseline Or SCr ≥354 µmol/L with an acute rise of ≥44 µmol/L in ≤24 hr Or Initiated on renal replacement therapy (irrespective of stage at time of initiation)	<0.3 mL/kg/hr for 24 hours Or Anuria for 12 hours

Source: Davenport et al. (2008); Murphy and Byrne (2010).

the day and therefore 24-hour urine collections may provide a better indicator of renal function than isolated blood samples. Furthermore, creatinine only reflects function at the ends of nephrons and thus provides a relatively late sign of dysfunction. In view of this, most laboratories now also routinely measure glomerular filtration rate (GFR), which is often estimated from creatinine levels. Normal GFR in the healthy adult is 90 mL/minute.

Indeed, in the scenario above, it is evident that John's urea and creatinine levels remained within the normal parameters and thus cannot be relied upon on their own as indicators of AKI. It is therefore important to recognize and be aware that the first sign of abnormality quite often is simply a reduction in urinary output. This is referred to as oliguria, which may be further defined as urinary output less than 0.5 mL/kg/body weight/hour (Davenport et al. 2008). In the case scenario here, it was noted that John's urinary output had reduced to 40 mL/hour. Given that John is 100 kg, he should therefore be producing at least 50 mL of urine per hour according to the calculation. In view of this, it was important that nursing staff were aware that this was a sign of deteriorating renal function and brought it to the doctor's attention as soon as possible. Unfortunately, however, consideration of urinary output according to body weight is not always carried out in practice and traditionally deterioration in urinary output was frequently not reported until the urine output was below 30 mL per hour. This would be adequate if patients weighed 60 kg or less, but the majority of patients falling into this weight range are increasingly uncommon (Woodrow 2009). Indeed, in the case of John, this is significantly less than it should be and waiting until his urinary output had fallen to this level before reporting it could result in an unacceptable delay in recognizing the condition. The scenario above does not specifically indicate the exact number of hours that John's urinary output remained at less than 0.5 mL/kg/hour. If this was the case for 6 hours,

John could be identified as being in the risk of AKI category as per the RIFLE guidelines or stage 1 as per the AKIN criteria. However, if the urinary output remained less than this for 12 hours, John could be identified as having now developed kidney injury or stage 2 AKI according to the AKIN guidelines.

2 **What factors may have precipitated acute kidney injury (AKI) in this particular patient?**

A The causes of AKI are most often categorized into three types, namely: volume-responsive or pre-renal, intra-renal (intrinsic) and post-renal. An overview of each of these types is useful to consider in order to fully appreciate why AKI may have occurred in this particular scenario.

TYPES OF AKI

Volume-responsive or pre-renal AKI

The biggest cause of volume-responsive or pre-renal AKI is impaired renal perfusion. The kidney is a very vascular organ and requires about 25% of cardiac output in order to function adequately. To maintain perfusion and function, the kidney autoregulates to maintain a continuous renal blood flow (Murphy and Byrne 2010). However, when the mean arterial blood pressure falls below 70 mmHg, the kidney's ability to autoregulate its own blood flow decreases (Byrne and Murphy 2008). There are various conditions that can lead to hypoperfusion, all of which can result in pre-renal failure but inadequate blood flow is usually caused by systemic hypotension due to hypovolaemia and/or cardiac failure (Woodrow 2009). In this particular scenario, it is evident that John experienced some degree of hypovolaemia with a 2-litre blood loss in theatre and therefore this is likely to be the main cause of his AKI. If the hypovolaemia is rapidly reversed by correction of the underlying cause, damage to the glomeruli and renal tubules can be avoided. In this case, it is apparent that some attempt was made to treat this volume-responsive or pre-renal AKI with fluid replacement therapy in theatre; however, this may not have been adequate as his urinary output has not returned to normal.

Intrinsic AKI

The term intrinsic renal failure refers to actual damage to renal cells such as the glomeruli and nephrons. This is more commonly referred to as acute tubular necrosis (ATN). Damage can be caused by inflammation and nephrotoxicity but more often occurs from ischaemia due to inadequate or delayed treatment of volume-responsive AKI thereby resulting in decreased blood flow to the kidneys (Woodrow 2009; Murphy and Byrne 2010). In John's case, it would appear that he did not receive adequate fluid replacement in theatre as alluded to above and therefore it is very likely that this could have resulted in prolonged hypoperfusion of the kidney and perhaps even have led to ATN. As noted by Woodrow (2009), even one night of unresolved volume-responsive AKI can be sufficient to cause ATN. Another possible reason that John may have developed AKI could be his past and current medication history. Many drugs, such as ACE inhibitors and NSAIDs, both of which John was prescribed, can destroy epithelial cells in the nephrons and lead to ATN of a toxic origin (Perkins and Kisiel 2005). Other causes of nephrotoxic ATN include antibiotics such as gentamicin, radiocontrast dye and also haemoglobin as a result of an incompatible blood transfusion (Murphy and Byrne 2010). There is no evidence from this scenario that John was administered the drugs mentioned above or that the blood transfusion received was incompatible; however, it is useful to be aware of their possible links to ATN. Intrinsic renal failure is more serious than pre-renal failure as it is not immediately reversible and will develop initially, despite addressing the underlying cause. In fact, it is suggested that intrinsic AKI will persist until the tissue damage resolves which can take typically 7–21 days (Perkins and Kisiel 2005).

Post-renal failure

Post-renal failure is the final type of AKI. It is caused by an obstruction to the flow of urine and this obstruction can occur anywhere between the renal tubules and the urethral outlet. Both intrinsic and extrinsic factors can cause this obstruction. Intrinsic factors include renal calculi or tumours and extrinsic factors include a surrounding or infiltrating tumour, for example, as a result of prostatic carcinoma, or a large inflammatory abdominal aortic aneurysm or even more simply may occur due to prostatic enlargement (Murphy and Byrne 2010). Given John's age, it is possible that he may have some degree of prostatic enlargement. However, overall, these post-renal causes do not appear to be the most likely reason for the development of AKI in this particular case scenario. Indeed, the overall incidence of this classification of AKI is estimated as being approximately 5–10% of cases (Byrne and Murphy 2008).

Other general criteria that increase the risk associated with developing AKI include if you are an older adult and have a long-term health problem such as diabetes, high blood pressure, heart failure or obesity and/or are already very ill in the hospital or in ICU (Ronco et al. 2009). Given that John is 72 years old and has a history of both diabetes and hypertension, he was already more susceptible to AKI notwithstanding the other contributing factors identified above.

3 | **Outline the key nursing care requirements that should now be considered in view of John's decline in his post-operative urine output measurements.**

A) If volume-responsive or pre-renal AKI is detected and managed by early intervention, intrinsic renal failure, which causes structural damage to the kidney, can be prevented from occurring (Davies 2009). In view of this, the first priority in the management of AKI is to obtain as accurate and comprehensive an assessment as possible to help establish whether or not John has AKI. In particular, the focus should be on urinary output along with fluid balance.

Monitor fluid balance

As already mentioned, a reduced urine output of less than 0.5 mL/kg body weight/hour is often the first indication of AKI, therefore the nurse must carefully consider John's urinary pattern and establish how much urine has passed and how long it has been less than 50 mL an hour (since John is 100 kg). It is also important to review the fluid balance chart to try to ascertain if the patient has received adequate fluid resuscitation. With a patient such as John who has had surgery, it is vital that this check includes the intra- and post-operative records in both the nursing and medical notes to establish how much blood or fluid was lost and exactly how much and what type of fluid was replaced. This knowledge of a patient's volume status is vital to determine whether he/she is hypovolaemic or indeed hypervolaemic (Murphy and Byrne 2010).

Consider fluid challenge

A major cause of pre-renal AKI is hypovolaemia and indeed this is likely to be the main cause of AKI in the case of John. In view of this, correction of any volume deficit is a key priority (Byrne and Murphy 2008). As noted by Osorio (2010), in the majority of cases, AKI can be resolved by adequate fluid challenge or replacement. A fluid challenge can be defined as a technique in which a large volume of fluid is administered over a defined period of time and the patient's response is closely observed. This is usually approximately 500 mL of crystalloid or colloid fluid given over 30 minutes (Dellinger et al. 2008). It is often argued whether colloids or crystalloids are better for the correction of hypovolaemia; however, Perel and Roberts (2007) in a Cochrane Review concluded that there is no real difference in patient outcome between the two fluids. The key factor is to replace lost volume.

Monitor BP and vital signs

It is also vital to monitor John's blood pressure and ascertain what the mean arterial pressure (MAP) is. Any alterations in blood pressure may indicate a reduction in intravascular volume and thus adequate renal perfusion pressures may not be maintained. It is estimated that a mean arterial blood pressure (MABP) of 80 mmHg may be required in the elderly and the hypertensive patient in particular to maintain sufficient perfusion and function of the kidney (Davies 2009). As John is 72 years old and has a known history of hypertension, it is therefore particularly important that the blood pressure is carefully considered in this case. Close monitoring of John's oxygen saturation levels would also be useful as maintaining oxygenation of renal cells is essential to prevent ischaemic damage from occurring (Perkins and Kisiel 2005). Signs of respiratory distress such as increased respiratory rate should also be observed particularly following fluid challenges as this may be indicative of fluid overload. Other presentation features of fluid overload or pulmonary oedema as a consequence of this include jugular venous distension, rapid pulse, hypertension and pitting oedema and thus vital signs must be monitored frequently (Murphy and Byrne 2010).

Monitor urine and electrolytes

Ward urinalysis is probably the most frequent urological investigation in hospitals but it is also useful for monitoring renal function. Indeed, it is now recommended that all patients presenting with AKI should have appropriate baseline investigations carried out including a urinalysis (Lewington and Kanagasundaram 2010). Positive protein values on reagent strip testing indicate intrinsic glomerular disease. Protein is not normally filtered by the glomerulus so proteinuria usually indicates an inflammatory response caused by disease that has allowed protein to pass through. Indeed, proteinuria has been identified as one of the most important indicators of kidney injury (Woodrow 2009). The presence of haematuria may also be suggestive of a lower urinary tract obstruction and often occurs in association with tumours and less commonly with calculi or infections (Lewington and Kanagasundaram 2010).

Frequent review of the patient's electrolyte levels, in particular the serum urea, creatinine and potassium levels are also required to ascertain what stage AKI the patient might be in and to monitor for hyperkalaemia. Hyperkalaemia is associated with decreased kidney regulation and consequently will effect potassium excretion. This can be very serious as it may lead to dysrhythmias which could result in cardiac arrest (Woodrow 2009).

Review medications

It is also important to carry out a review of the patient's medications when AKI is considered and any nephrotoxic agents should be discontinued where possible, unless contraindicated. John is currently prescribed ACE inhibitors and NSAIDs, both of which are known to be particularly nephrotoxic (Byrne and Murphy 2008) and therefore will need to be reviewed. It is also important to be aware there is no specific pharmacological therapy proven to effectively treat AKI secondary to hypoperfusion injury and/or sepsis (Lewington and Kanagasundaram 2010). In fact, it is now established that the historical practice of giving loop diuretics, such as furosemide to treat AKI is dangerous and is not advocated by the UK Renal Association in the deterrence and treatment of AKI (Davenport et al. 2008). In volume-responsive AKI, if diuretics are given, they will actually worsen hypovolaemia and consequently hasten ATN, thereby increasing mortality. Furthermore, although they may result in more urine being produced, it is likely to be of poor quality since it does not remove waste products adequately and therefore does not resolve the problem (Woodrow 2009). In view of this, it is useful to ensure that John is not currently prescribed or receiving diuretic therapy.

Later that night, John's urinary output was noted to be less than 20 mL/hour. His blood results are also as follows:

Sodium: 134 mmol/L (135–145 mmol/L)
Potassium: 5.7 mmol/L (3.4–5.1 mmol/L)
Urea: 12.1 mmol/L (1.7–8.3 mmol/L)
Creatinine: 215 μmol/L (female 50–90 μmol/L, male 70–120 μmol/L)
Calcium: 2.4 mmol/L (2.2–2.5 mmol/L).

It is therefore apparent that his condition is deteriorating. He has also started to complain of a metallic taste in his mouth.

4   **The serum potassium level is now elevated. Discuss the treatment that John should receive for this.**

A   John's serum potassium has now risen to 5.7 mmol/litre. This has the potential to be life-threatening as hyperkalaemia can cause cardiac arrhythmias. It would therefore be useful to attach John to a cardiac monitor and observe for signs of peaked T waves or indeed any arrhythmias (Davies 2009). When potassium levels are above 5.5 mmol/litre, as they are in this case, treatment also needs to be initiated. The most common first-line therapy for the management of hyperkalaemia is an intravenous insulin and dextrose infusion. This treatment forces potassium out of the blood into the cells for a few hours thereby temporarily reducing the levels in the blood (Mahoney et al. 2005). During this infusion, it is vital that John's blood sugars are monitored closely as there is the potential for patients to become hypoglycaemic due to the insulin administration (Murphy and Byrne 2010). Evidence from the Cochrane database also states that nebulised salbutamol is another useful first-line therapy for hyper-kalaemia. Furthermore, it is suggested that when used in combination with an insulin and glucose infusion, the results may be even more effective especially when the hyperkalaemia is severe (Mahoney et al. 2005). Salbutamol nebulisers can, however, cause palpitations and therefore, if given, John will need to have his heart rate and rhythm monitored closely (Davies 2009). Calcium gluconate or calcium resonium may also be given to treat hyperkalaemia; however, neither tends to have a long-lasting effect and therefore tend not to be used as frequently as the other therapies (Perkins and Kisiel 2005; Davies 2009). Potassium should also be restricted in John's diet and therefore a dietician referral may be useful. Finally, the potassium levels should continue to be monitored closely to ensure that treatment is effective. However, if the patient has a refractory hyperkalaemia >6.5 mmol/litre, renal replacement therapy should be initiated (Davenport et al. 2008).

5   **John's urea levels are also rising. What effects might high urea levels have on John?**

A   The symptoms of uraemia (high urea levels) can cause the patient to experience a distorted sense of taste, known as dysgeusia, which can result in a metallic taste in the mouth, as experienced by John. This can be extremely unpleasant for the patient and may cause the patient to experience nausea or vomiting which must be addressed (Murphy and Byrne 2010). If uraemic products were to accumulate further, this can cause uraemic syndrome which has the potential to be life-threatening as one of its most serious consequences is interference with the clotting cascade. This can expose the patient to bleeding tendencies which could poten-tially lead to severe and uncontrolled bleeding (Osorio 2010). Another consequence of uraemic syndrome may be the development of intractable hiccups. This may require manage-ment by dialysis if it were to persist (Murphy and Byrne 2010).

Overall it was felt that John had developed AKI as he was not given adequate fluids to prevent volume-responsive AKI following his surgery. Further fluids have since been prescribed and John's NSAIDs have been stopped at present. An insulin and dextrose infusion was also prescribed to treat his hyperkalaemia. His electrolyte levels are now showing signs of returning to normal and the urinary output is beginning to increase. It is now hoped that the AKI is resolving and no further intervention such as renal replacement therapy will be required.

6 **Why is it important to keep monitoring the urine output closely now that John appears to be recovering?**

A It is important to continue to be vigilant with regard to urinary output at this stage as one of the first signs of improvement of AKI may be a diuretic phase. The diuretic or polyuric phase is marked by urine output that can range from normal (1–2 litres/day) to as high as 6–8 litres/day and is accompanied by significant losses of potassium, sodium and water (Redmond et al. 2004). This is a sign of recovery and that the tubular cells are beginning to regenerate. However, initially these cells are immature and therefore do not usually function effectively. Consequently, although filtration improves, tubular reabsorption and solute exchange are inadequate, causing large volumes of poor quality urine, and serum urea and creatinine levels remain high (Woodrow 2009). During this phase it is therefore important that the nurse closely assesses the patient's fluid balance and electrolyte levels. Fluid intake may need to be increased to account for the fluid volume lost and electrolytes such as sodium and potassium levels corrected. The patient should also be observed for signs of dehydration such as loss of skin elasticity and a dry mouth (Murphy and Byrne 2010). The recovery phase is reached when tubular function has restored and the urinary output, and urea and creatinine levels have returned to normal again. However, it can sometimes take 6 months to a year for full regeneration of tubular tissues, before the tubular cells begin to perform as effectively as they should and renal function is fully restored (Perkins and Kisiel 2005). In view of this, the patient needs to be aware of the importance of reporting any further problems with urinary output in a timely manner.

Key points

- Acute kidney injury has replaced the term acute renal failure and can be categorized into three types: volume-responsive (pre-renal) AKI, intra-renal (intrinsic) AKI, and post-renal AKI.
- Early detection and management of volume-responsive AKI are vital to prevent intrinsic renal failure and thus structural damage to the kidney occurring.
- Close ongoing monitoring of urinary output is vital in the recovery phase as it is frequently accompanied by a significant diuretic phase.

REFERENCES

Bellomo, R., Ronco, C., Kellum, J.A., Mehta, R.L., Palevsky, P., and the AADQI Workgroup (2004) Acute renal failure – definition, outcome measures, animal models, fluid therapy and information technology needs: the second International Consensus Conference of the Acute Dialysis Quality Initiative Workgroup, *Critical Care*, 8(4): R204–R212.

Byrne, G. and Murphy, F. (2008) Acute kidney injury and its impact on the cardiac patient, *British Journal of Cardiac Nursing*, 3(9): 416–22.

Davenport, A., Kanagasundaram, S., Lewington, A. and Stevens, P. (2008) *UK Renal Association Clinical Practice Guidelines: Acute Kidney Injury*. London: UK Renal Association. Available at: http://www.renal.org/guidelines/module5.html (accessed 24 October 2011).

Davies, A. (2009) Diagnosing and classifying acute kidney injury, *Journal of Renal Nursing*, 1(1): 9–12.

Dellinger, R.P., Levy, M.M., Carlet, J.M., Bion, J., Parker, M.M., Jaeschke, R. et al. (2008) Surviving Sepsis Campaign: International Surviving Sepsis Campaign Guidelines Committee: international guidelines for management of severe sepsis and septic shock, *Critical Care Medicine*, 36(1): 296–327.

Lewington, A. and Kanagasundaram, S. (2010) *Clinical Practice Guidelines: Acute Kidney Injury*. Available at: www.renal.org/guidelines (accessed 22 October 2011).

Mahoney, B.A., Smith, W.A.D., Lo, D., Tsoi, K., Tonelli, M. and Clase, C. (2005) Emergency interventions for hyperkalaemia, *The Cochrane Collaboration Cochrane Reviews*. Available at: http://www.cochrane.org/reviews/en/ab00567.html (accessed 24 October 2011).

Murphy, F. and Byrne, G. (2010) The role of the nurse in the management of acute kidney injury, *British Journal of Nursing*, 19(3): 146–52.

Osorio, C. (2010) Renal assessment and support, in F. Creed and C. Spiers (eds) *Care of the Acutely Ill Adult*. Oxford: Oxford University Press.

Perel, P. and Roberts, I.G. (2007) Colloids versus crystalloids for fluid resuscitation in critically ill patients, *The Cochrane Collaboration Cochrane Reviews*. Available at: http://www.cochrane.org/reviews/en/ab000567.htm (accessed 24 October 2011).

Perkins, C., Kisiel, M. (2005) Utilizing physiological knowledge to care for acute renal failure, *British Journal of Nursing*, 14(14): 768–73.

Redmond, A., McDevitt, M. and Barnes, S. (2004) Acute renal failure: recognition and treatment in ward patients, *Nursing Standard*, 11(18): 46–53.

Ronco, C., Bellomo, R. and Kellum, J.A. (2009) *Critical Care Nephrology*, 2nd edn. Philadelphia, PA: Saunders Elsevier.

Woodrow, P. (2009) Acute kidney injury, in T. Moore and P. Woodrow (eds) *High Dependency Nursing Care: Observation, Intervention and Support for Level 2 Patients*. Abingdon: Routledge.

PART 4
Neurological System

CASE STUDY 7
Head injury
Aidín McKinney

Case outline

James is a student in his mid-twenties. He had been out for the night with a few friends during which he consumed copious amounts of alcohol. Later on he was found in an unconscious state by some passers-by who called for an ambulance. He was brought to A&E where he has since regained some level of consciousness but is unable to provide a very coherent history. His Glasgow Coma Scale is 13 and a laceration has been noted to the back of his head, with some swelling now also evident.

---

1 **Reflect on the scenario above and consider the immediate action that needs to be taken.**

A As James's level of consciousness is reduced, it is first of all imperative that the immediate action to be considered should be the maintenance of a patent airway (Cree 2003). In the unconscious or semi-conscious patient, obstruction most commonly occurs at the level of the pharynx and occurs due to the reduced muscle tone that causes the tongue to fall back and occlude the airway (Resuscitation Council 2006). As James has been drinking, he is also at risk of aspirating gastric contents through vomiting. Immediate action that can be used to maintain a clear airway include head tilt, chin lift or if the patient has a suspected cervical spine injury, jaw thrust should be carried out (Resuscitation Council (UK) 2006).

A full ABCDE assessment should then be conducted, including the Glasgow Coma Scale.

2 **How would you assess James using the Glasgow Coma Scale?**

A The Glasgow Coma Scale (GCS) is an internationally recognized tool which is used to assess the conscious level of the patient. It is based on three behaviours: best eye, best verbal and best motor responses (see Table 7.1). Correct assessment and recording of these will detect if the patient's condition is improving, stabilizing or deteriorating. However, it is proposed that the GCS is not always used accurately in practice (May 2009). It is suggested that there is a possibility of different interpretations of Glasgow Coma Scale values particularly if staff use a variety of painful stimuli or reaction-to-light methods when carrying out the assessment. A uniform way of carrying out the GCS is therefore essential to provide the most accurate assessment of the patient's neurological status (Waterhouse 2009).

Table 7.1 Main observations on patient with a head injury

Observations	Indications
Pupil size and reactivity	Abnormal pupil size and response are an indication of raised intracranial pressure (ICP). This may be due to swelling, a bleed or perhaps a haematoma (Dawes et al. 2007). Pupil constriction and dilation are controlled by the third cranial nerve or the oculomotor nerve. Pressure on this nerve will produce sluggish, unequal or suddenly dilated pupils. These are indicators of deterioration and require urgent medical attention (Cree 2003). For example, a unilateral dilated pupil may indicate brain herniation or raised ICP and fixed pupils may indicate severe mid-brain damage (Dawes et al. 2007). It is also useful to be aware that certain drugs such as atropine dilate the pupil while opiates constrict the pupil (Edwards 2001)
Limb movements	Assessment of limb responses provide information about motor function and any deficiencies may indicate a developing weakness or loss of movement caused by raised ICP. It is important to assess and record each limb separately (Dawes et al. 2007)
Respiratory rate	The autonomic respiratory control centres are located in the pons and upper medulla of the brainstem. Increased ICP can put pressure on these areas and therefore can lead to respiratory changes, including changes to breathing patterns such as Cheyne-Stokes respiration (rapid rhythmic breathing with periods of apnoea). When abnormal respiration is combined with hypertension and bradycardia, this is called Cushing's triad which is a late sign of brainstem dysfunction and is often accompanied by cerebral herniation which results in brainstem death (Suadoni 2009)
Heart rate	The control centres for heart rate and indeed blood pressure and respiration are all located in the brainstem. Therefore any increased pressure to these areas can affect their control (Edwards 2001). In early stages of increasing ICP, the pulse rate tends to remain relatively stable; however, in later stages bradycardia is often observed (Suadoni 2009)
Blood pressure	It is essential that the blood pressure is monitored closely in the head injury patient. Hypotension can result in an associated drop in cerebral perfusion pressure (CPP), leading to ischaemia. Normally the brain can autoregulate, which is the ability to maintain stable cerebral blood flow irrespective of changes in systemic blood pressure. Thus, if the blood pressure increases, cerebral blood vessels will constrict and vice versa. However, in head injury patients, the ability to autoregulate may become impaired, and cerebral blood flow becomes 'pressure passive' and is directly influenced by systemic blood pressure. A CPP of 60–70 mmHg is recommended to provide adequate cerebral blood flow (CBF) (McLeod 2004a). CPP is the difference between the systemic mean arterial pressure and the ICP. In areas where ICP is not directly monitored, mean arterial pressure (MAP) should be maintained above 80–90 mmHg in order to maintain adequate CPP (Cree 2003). In the early stages of rising ICP, blood pressure is likely to remain quite stable. However, in the later stages, increased ICP reduces CPP. This will

eventually activate the ischaemic reflex leading to vasoconstriction and a consequent rise in blood pressure. This in turn will cause vagal stimulation which will decrease heart rate in an effort to reduce the blood pressure. This combination of hypertension and bradycardia is therefore characteristically seen in patients with significant rises in ICP and is quite a concerning sign (Suadoni 2009)

Temperature	Body temperature is controlled by the hypothalamus. Thus fluctuations or increases in body temperature may indicate damage to the hypothalamus caused by raised ICP. A raised temperature also increases cerebral metabolic oxygen requirements and when oxygenation of the brain may already be reduced it is another unwanted complication (Edwards 2001). However, it is also important for the nurse to ascertain if the hyperthermia is caused by the raised ICP or is due to an infection (Suadoni 2009)
Blood oxygen saturations	If the oxygen content of blood falls, the cerebral blood flow will increase in an effort to maintain cerebral oxygenation. This too will increase ICP (McLeod 2004b).Oxygen saturations should be monitored continually and oxygen therapy should be administered to maintain saturations above 98% to reduce the risk of secondary brain injury that can result as a consequence of hypoxaemia (McLeod 2004a)

BEST RESPONSES

Best eye-opening response

The patient is considered to have spontaneous eye opening when the eyes are open without the need for any stimulation by the healthcare professional. If the eyes are closed, their state of arousal can then be assessed by the degree of stimulation that is required to get them to open their eyes, i.e. to speech or pain (Edwards 2001; Palmer and Knight 2006). When trying to elicit a response to speech, Waterhouse (2009) suggests that asking a patient a question such as if they 'want a cup of tea' can more often achieve a better response than simply calling the patient's name and asking them to open their eyes. If there is still no response, then a deeper stimulus is required, the intensity of which should be gradually increased. Unfortunately there would appear to be many different variations in the type of painful stimuli that are used in practice and this may account for some of the inaccuracies in the GCS. Painful stimuli generally fall into two categories: central and peripheral. It has been suggested that to assess eye opening, a peripheral painful stimuli should be used rather than a central one. This is because central pain is often said to cause eye closure by inducing a grimacing effect (Iankova 2006).

Application of peripheral pain should be carried out by applying direct pressure at the side of the finger for approximately 10–15 seconds (Waterhouse 2009). Pressure should not be applied directly onto the nail bed as it could cause damage to the structures just under the nail bed and may lead to bruising due to capillary damage (Edwards 2001).

The patient should respond by opening their eyes to inspect the source of injury or to identify the perpetrator and may also attempt to move the limb away from the pain (Waterhouse 2009).

Best verbal response

The best verbal response assesses both comprehension or understanding of what has been said and ability to express thoughts into words. A person who is orientated should know their name, where they are and the time of day. If these are answered correctly, then the patient is said to be orientated. It is not necessary to ask the patient the day of the week, date or year (Edwards 2001). As John has been drinking alcohol, it may be more difficult to assess his 'best verbal' response because alcohol causes cognitive impairment and thus affects both intellectual and linguistic ability. Thus, intoxicated patients such as John may well be confused, use inappropriate words or even make inappropriate sounds. It is therefore particularly challenging for healthcare professionals to accurately identify if reduced consciousness levels are caused by the head injury or by the alcohol alone (Edwards 2001). However, brain injury should always be suspected as being the primary cause of altered consciousness and reduced GCS until a significant brain injury has been fully assessed and excluded (Iankova 2006; NICE 2007).

Best motor response

A lack of motor response also points to deterioration in the functional state of the brain as it indicates that the patient is not as able to process sensory input or motor activity (Iankova 2006). When assessing 'best motor response', it is recommended that the patient is asked to 'put out your tongue' or 'hold up two fingers' to assess their ability to obey simple commands. Edwards (2001) states that these are preferable to asking the patient to 'squeeze my fingers' as this is a primitive reflex and thus may occur involuntarily and not in response to a command. If the patient does not obey simple commands, a painful stimulus must be applied. When assessing the patient's ability to localize to pain, a central painful stimulus should be applied (Dawes et al. 2007).

Application of central pain. It has been proposed that the three most common ways to apply a central painful stimulus in practice are by the trapezium squeeze, the supraorbital pressure and the sternal rub. Of these, a number of articles highlight that the sternal rub should no longer be advocated since it can lead to bruising upon the patient's chest (Edwards 2001; Dawes et al. 2007; Waterhouse 2009). Unfortunately this practice still seems to occur despite it being strongly discouraged. The aim of applying painful stimuli is to assess the depth of coma, not to cause long-term or unnecessary pain or damage. Use of the supra-orbital pressure stimulus should also be avoided if the patient has sustained any head or facial trauma (Dawes et al. 2007). Thus, it would appear that the trapezius squeeze may be the most appropriate stimulus to use when head injury is suspected. Painful stimuli should be applied in a careful manner and for no longer than 30 seconds (Edwards 2001).

3 What vital observations also need to be carried out (and how often)? Discuss the significance of measuring these in a head injury patient.

A NICE (2007) emphasizes that for patients admitted for head injury observation, the minimum acceptable neurological observations that need to be documented in addition to the GCS are: pupil size and reactivity, limb movements, respiratory rate, heart rate, blood pressure, temperature and blood oxygen saturations. NICE (2007) also advocates that these observations should be performed and recorded half-hourly until a GCS equal to 15 has been achieved. Once a GCS of 15 has been achieved, observations should then be carried out half-hourly for 2 hours, then 1-hourly for 4 hours and then 2-hourly thereafter. However, should the patient's condition deteriorate again, observations should then revert back to half-hourly.

> Following an initial assessment, James was admitted to a medical ward overnight for observation. By the early hours of the morning, James suddenly became unresponsive to verbal stimulation and his breathing became more laboured.

4 What could have contributed to the deterioration in James's condition?

A It is likely that James's intracranial pressure (ICP) has now risen which has led to this deterioration in his condition. ICP is the pressure exerted by the intracranial contents against the skull. The skull is a rigid structure that is made up of three compartments: the brain tissue (80%), blood (10%) and cerebrospinal fluid (CSF) (10%). The Monroe-Kellie doctrine states that should there be an increase in one of these compartments, there must be a reciprocal decrease in one of the other two compartments otherwise the ICP will increase (McLeod 2004b). A normal ICP is 0–10 mmHg and increased ICP is a sustained elevation in pressure above 15 mmHg. The most common cause of increased ICP is cerebral oedema. This is said to occur between 1–18 hours after head trauma and quite often the volume peaks at day 3 (May 2009). As the swelling increases, the skull is unable to cope with the increased volume and therefore the ICP rises. When the ICP rises, certain compensatory mechanisms come into play in an effort to reduce the risk of herniation or brainstem injury occurring. According to the Monroe-Kellie doctrine, brain tissue is least able to compensate for this change in volume, so movement of CSF and cerebral blood flow is most likely to occur. However, this redistribution of CSF and cerebral blood flow does not really solve the problem as cerebral blood flow limitation results in cerebral ischaemia. The body will try to further compensate for the decrease in cerebral perfusion pressure by raising the blood pressure and dilating the brain's blood vessels. This will result in an increase in the cerebral blood volume. However, this will also lower the cerebral perfusion pressure further, thus causing a vicious cycle (McLeod 2004b). It is estimated that patients with normal blood pressure can retain normal alertness with an ICP of 25–40 mmHg. However, when the ICP exceeds this, the cerebral perfusion pressure falls to a level that results in a loss of consciousness (May 2009). It would seem that John's ICP level is significantly high to lead to his reduction in consciousness level.

5   **What nursing interventions need to be considered in order to reduce the risk of ICP rising any higher?**

A   When a patient has been admitted with a head injury, the goal of the treatment is to stabilize them and to prevent further or secondary injury from occurring. Primary injury is the damage that occurs at the time of the actual event and is unavoidable. Secondary injury, however, may occur any time after the initial injury and may be preventable, mainly by trying to ensure that neuronal hypoxia and hypoperfusion do not occur (Garner and Amin 2007).

When the ICP is raised, the nurses' main goals are to monitor and manage the existing patient's condition and ICP, but also to consider nursing activities that will minimize the risk of ICP levels rising any higher. Some of these key activities will now be considered.

NURSING INTERVENTIONS

Maintain blood pressure

Hypotension can have a detrimental effect on patient outcome due to the associated fall that occurs in CPP. For this reason it is recommended that in areas where ICP is not directly monitored, the mean arterial pressure should be maintained above 80–90 mmHg to maintain adequate CPP. This should first of all be maintained by ensuring that the patient is adequately hydrated. When giving fluids, however, solutions containing dextrose should be avoided as they tend to decrease plasma osmolality to increase brain water content (Garner and Amin 2007). Therefore this can lead to an increase in cerebral oedema and ischaemia by increasing the osmotic pressure. Glucose is also easily converted to lactate in hypoxic states, producing an acidosis. Where blood pressure needs to be manipulated with inotropes, the patient will require even closer monitoring and thus may need to be cared for in an intensive care setting (Cree 2003).

Control of oxygen/carbon dioxide levels

Alterations in respiratory gases can have an effect on cerebral blood vessels and therefore cerebral blood flow (CBF). If the PaO_2 falls below 6.7 kPa, vasodilation causes the CBF to increase in an effort to maintain cerebral oxygenation. This too will lead to an increase in ICP. Raised carbon dioxide levels also cause a vasodilatory effect and therefore will again lead to a rise in ICP. For this reason, normocapnia, or normal $PaCO_2$ levels, is recommended (Garner and Amin 2007).

Nutrition and blood sugar control

Head injury induces a state of hypermetabolism and hypercatabolism and thereby increases the demands of the brain for oxygen and glucose. This increases the cerebral blood volume and hence ICP. It is therefore recommended that where normal oral intake is not feasible, early enteral feeding is commenced as soon as possible. This also encourages normal gut peristalsis and discourages the translocation of bacteria (Mestecky 2006). Blood glucose levels should also be maintained within normal limits. As noted by McLeod (2004b), glucose is metabolized to carbon dioxide and water, thus an excess of these could cause cerebral oedema, increasing ICP.

Positioning

Careful positioning of head-injured patients can be very important in maintaining ICP control. In particular it is recommended that patients with raised ICP are routinely cared for with their heads elevated to 30 degrees. It is suggested that this method facilitates the drainage of venous blood from the brain and may also move CSF from the cranial to the spinal subarachnoid space (Fan 2004). It is also suggested that neck rotation and head flexion should be avoided as they can increase ICP because drainage of fluid from the brain is impeded (Cree 2003).

Bowel management

Constipation will not only cause patient discomfort but will also increase intra-abdominal pressure. Raised intra-abdominal pressure increases intrathoracic pressure which in turn will increase ICP. Straining at stool will also increase ICP, thus a bowel management programme should be initiated as soon as possible, including being cognisant of monitoring fluid levels and analgesia such as opioids. It is also recommended that stool softeners are administered and enemas avoided as these may increase intra-abdominal pressure (McLeod 2004b).

Temperature regulation

Hyperthermia in patients with head injury increases the cerebral metabolic rate. Indeed, it is suggested that each one degree rise in core temperature is associated with a 7% increase in cerebral metabolism. Hyperpyrexias should therefore be controlled with antipyretic agents, such as paracetamol and passive cooling methods such as tepid sponging (Garner and Amin 2007).

Clustering of activities

Many nursing interventions such as repositioning, personal care and suctioning when carried out in close succession can have a cumulative effect on increasing ICP. Thus clustering of activities should be minimized as much as possible (Suadoni 2009).

Eventually James's GCS fell to 8 and he was almost unresponsive. His family have arrived at the ward. They are extremely anxious and distressed and are demanding to see James.

6 **What should the ward nurse now do once a further deterioration in GCS has been noted?**

A Patients with a GCS of 8 or less should be intubated to protect the airway. The nurse needs to alert medical staff immediately, including the anaesthetist. The Intensive Care Unit (ICU) needs to be informed and an ICU bed arranged. Family also need to be informed regarding the deterioration in James's condition (Cree 2003).

7 **Discuss whether the family members should be allowed to visit James.**

A NICE (2007) and the Department of Health (2001) promote the involvement of families in the recovery and rehabilitation of head injury patients. It is suggested that when a good relationship between the patient and relatives exists, involvement in the patient's care should be encouraged because ICP is thought to be considerably reduced in the presence of familiar voices and touch (Odell 1996; Cree 2003). Thus relatives should be encouraged to talk and make physical contact with the head-injured patient (such as by holding hands). However, NICE (2007) also highlight that relatives should not feel obliged to do so and indeed if they wish to spend time with the patient, they should be reminded to take regular breaks. Care should also be taken to ensure that upsetting conversations such as discussions about prognosis do not take place over the patient as it may cause emotional distress and increase ICP. Thus, even if a patient is comatose, family members should be advised to assume that the patient can hear and understand all that is being said (Suadoni 2009). In the case of James's relatives, it is therefore important that they are first spoken to away from the patient and given information about his condition and given an opportunity to vent their distress before visiting. NICE (2007) also recommend that information sheets detailing the nature of head injury and any investigations likely to be used should be made available.

Key points

- The Glasgow Coma Scale (GCS) is the internationally recognized tool which is used to assess the conscious level of the patient.
- Patients with a GCS of 8 or less should be intubated to protect the airway.
- If a patient is comatose, family members should be advised to assume that the patient can hear and understand all that is being said.

REFERENCES

Cree, C. (2003) Acquired brain injury: acute management, *Nursing Standard*, 18(11): 45–54.

Dawes, E., Lloyd, H. and Durham, L. (2007) Monitoring and recording patients' neurological observations, *Nursing Standard*, 22(10): 40–5.

Department of Health (2001) *Government Response to the Health Select Committee: Inquiry into Head Injury Rehabilitation*. Available at: www.doh.gov.uk/head-injuries/ (accessed February 2011).

Edwards, S.L. (2001) Using the Glasgow Coma Scale: analysis and limitations, *British Journal of Nursing*, 10(2): 92–101.

Fan, J.Y. (2004) Effect of backrest position on intracranial pressure and cerebral perfusion pressure in individuals with brain injury: a systematic review, *Journal of Neuroscience Nursing*, 36(5): 278–88.

Garner, A. and Amin, Y. (2007) The management of raised intracranial pressure: a multidisciplinary approach, *British Journal of Neuroscience Nursing*, 3(11): 516–21.

Iankova, A. (2006) The Glasgow Coma Scale: clinical application in Emergency departments, *Emergency Nurse*, 14(8): 30–5.

May, K. (2009) The pathophysiology and causes of raised intracranial pressure, *British Journal of Nursing*, 18(15): 911–14.

McLeod, A. (2004a) Traumatic injuries to the head and spine 1: mechanisms of injury, *British Journal of Nursing*, 13(16): 940–7.

McLeod, A. (2004b) Traumatic injuries to the head and spine 2: nursing considerations, *British Journal of Nursing*, 13(17): 1041–9.

Mestecky, A. (2006) Metabolic responses after severe head injury and how to optimise nutrition: a literature review, *British Journal of Neuroscience Nursing*, 2(2): 73–9.

NICE (National Institute for Health and Clinical Excellence) (2007) *Head Injury: Triage, Assessment, Investigation and Early Management of Head Injury in Infants, Children and Adults*, Clinical Guideline No. 56. London: NICE.

Odell, M. (1996) Intracranial pressure monitoring: nursing in a district general hospital, *Nursing in Critical Care*, 1(5): 245–7.

Palmer, R. and Knight, J. (2006) Assessment of altered conscious level in clinical practice, *British Journal of Nursing*, 15(22): 1255–9.

Resuscitation Council (UK) (2006) *Advanced Life Support Manual*, 4th edn. London: Resuscitation Council.

Suadoni, M.T. (2009) Raised intracranial pressure: nursing observations and interventions, *Nursing Standard*, 23(43): 35–40.

Waterhouse, C. (2009) The use of painful stimulus in relation to Glasgow Coma Scale observations, *British Journal of Neuroscience Nursing*, 5(5): 209–14.

Acute stroke
Karen Page

Case outline

Margaret Smyth, a 56-year-old lady arrived at the A&E department of the hospital having experienced a sudden collapse while at home. She was found in the kitchen by a builder carrying out some repairs at the house. Since she was clearly unwell, he had called the emergency services immediately. Based on the use of the FAST assessment tool the paramedics had alerted A&E prior to her arrival as there was evidence that the patient might have suffered a stroke. Her husband has been informed of the situation by a neighbour and is en route to the hospital.

---

1 **Review the FAST assessment tool.**

A In patients with a sudden onset of neurological symptoms, a validated tool such as FAST should be used outside hospital to screen for a diagnosis of stroke or transient ischaemic attack (TIA). Stroke is now regarded as a medical emergency in which early intervention can have a vital role in reducing long-term disability and therefore healthcare staff and the general public should be educated to recognize possible signs and symptoms of a stroke. The FAST tool is a simple straightforward method of highlighting those patients who require urgent transfer to hospital (Harbinson et al. 2003).

Check point: FAST TEST – Face Arm Speech Test

F = **F**acial weakness – can the person smile? Has their mouth or eye drooped? Look for lack of symmetry.

A = **A**rm weakness – can the person raise both arms? Does one arm fall down or appear to be weaker than the other?

S = **S**peech problems – can the person speak clearly and understand what you say?

T = **T**est all three symptoms. If one or more is abnormal, suspect stroke.

Time to call 999.

On admission, Margaret is alert but visibly distressed and unable to communicate clearly with the staff due to the presence of dysarthria. She is also noted to have right-sided facial weakness.

A patient assessment revealed the following information:

Temperature: 37.2°C
Pulse: 88 beats per minute, regular
Respirations: 22 breaths per minute
B/P: 170/100 mmHg
O$_2$ Saturation: 95%
Blood sugar: 6.2 mmol/L
No major abnormalities are noted on the ECG.

Glasgow Coma Scale 15
Assessment of the patient establishes neurological deficits in sensory and motor responses in the right arm and leg resulting in hemiplegia and neglect of the right side.

Time of onset was established as less than one hour ago by information received from the ambulance personnel.

2   What additional tools can be used in the A&E unit to help establish a diagnosis of stroke?

A   Healthcare personnel who are working in A&E departments and other settings need to view patients with stroke as a medical emergency and ensure these patients are assessed rapidly using a validated tool such as ROSIER. These patients need to be identified early to qualify for thrombolytic therapy and other cost-effective diagnostic studies and interventions (Hinkle et al. 2007).

Check point: ROSIER – Recognition of Stroke in the Emergency Room

ROSIER is a seven-item clinical diagnostic stroke scale that is simple, sensitive, specific and suitable for use in the Accident and Emergency department. Factors assessed include problems with vision and speech, loss of consciousness and face, arm and/or leg weakness.

The scale includes questions to identify syncope and seizure which can mimic stroke symptoms and therefore has a high diagnostic sensitivity (Nor et al. 2005). It should be noted, however, that neither the FAST test nor the ROSIER scale are useful for predicting the symptoms of posterior stroke, which usually includes visual, balance or co-ordination problems (Lawson and Gibbons 2009).

3 **Outline the pathological processes that may result in a stroke.**

A During a stroke, parts of the brain are deprived of oxygen either because of the blockage of an artery due to the presence of a thrombus or embolism or as a result of a haemorrhage. Ischaemia is thought to account for approximately 85% of cases and primary haemorrhage for about 15% of presentations (Bath and Lees 2000).

Think

Thrombosis

Vessel occlusion arises from thrombi formed in the arteries supplying the brain or in the intracranial vessels as a result of atherosclerosis. In the cerebral circulation atherosclerotic plaques are found most commonly at arterial bifurcations or forks in the artery, e.g. the bifurcation of the internal carotid artery. Vessel occlusion can also arise from small vessel disease deep within the brain.

Embolus

Embolic stroke results from cerebral ischaemia secondary to blockage of the vessel by an embolus (McCance and Huether 2006). The most frequent site of embolic strokes is the middle cerebral artery, reflecting the large distribution of this vessel and its position as the terminus of the carotid artery. Various cardiac conditions predispose to the formation of emboli that produce embolic stroke including for example rheumatic heart disease, atrial fibrillation, or recent myocardial infarction (McCance and Huether 2006).

Haemorrhage

This occurs when a cerebral blood vessel ruptures and causes haemorrhage into the brain tissue – intracerebral haemorrhage. This results in direct neuronal injury from the pressure effects of the ensuing haematoma. The most common predisposing factor is hypertension; however, other causes include aneurysm, trauma, tumours, vascular malformations and illicit drug use (McCance and Huether 2006).

---

4 **Consider the nursing management of the clinical features highlighted in the assessment of this patient. Give a rationale for your answer.**

A Table 8.1 shows the nursing management of the clinical features of a stroke.

Table 8.1 Clinical features and nursing management of a stroke

Clinical features	Management and rationale
AIRWAY	
Assessment	*Management*
Margaret is alert though agitated and distressed with communication difficulties due to dysarthria	Reassure the patient that although you cannot always determine what she wishes to communicate, you will try to establish her queries/concerns and act accordingly. This is particularly important on admission, for example with respect to information regarding nursing and other interventions or elimination needs
	The use of non-verbal communication and open/closed questions will help to facilitate communication at this point
	Speak slowly and clearly and allow time for the patient to respond to you
	Avoid making assumptions and always try to confirm information with the patient
	Reassure the patient that her husband will arrive soon
	Do not assume the patient cannot understand what you are saying even if she has dysarthria
	Rationale
	Stroke has affected the patient's ability to clearly verbalize by causing injury in the left hemisphere which contains the area associated with speech – Broca's area. This means that the patient is unable to verbalize clearly
	Patients with dysarthria have functional limitations in speech intelligibility, rate and naturalness. There is no reason to suspect any impairment of understanding in a patient with dysarthria as would be the case with aphasia (Borthwick 2012) Communication difficulties can, however, cause severe distress and frustration when patients are unable to communicate their requests/concerns
	Management
Facial weakness	Keep patient nil by mouth until a swallowing assessment can be undertaken by trained personnel (usually a nurse) using a validated water swallow tool to assess whether or not the patient has a safe swallow
	Provide oral hygiene while the patient is nil by mouth (ISWP 2008; Kelly et al. 2010)
	If the patient is to receive thrombolytic therapy, they should be kept nil by mouth prior to and during administration and then assessed for swallowing ability as soon as possible (Soames and Bergman 2007)

If patient is nil by mouth, IV fluids will be required to maintain hydration; however, it is recommended to avoid the use of dextrose in the first 48 hours as this may mask other pathological changes (ISWP 2008)

Rationale

There is potential for the airway to be dysfunctional with a risk of aspiration following stroke as evidenced in Margaret's case by signs of facial weakness. Dysphagia is common in up to 50% of stroke patients (Rowat et al. 2009), therefore guidelines recommend that all stroke patients have a simple bedside swallow test performed by an appropriately trained person to identify those with swallowing difficulties (ISWP 2008; NICE 2008). This will guide future management of fluid and nutritional requirements for patients

BREATHING

Assessment

Oxygen saturation 95%
Respiratory rate 22
breaths per minute

Management

Monitor and record observations regularly as patient's condition requires for any change in respiratory rate/pattern and oxygen saturations
Position the patient to maximize chest expansion

Patients with a stroke should receive supplemental oxygen only if their oxygen saturations drop below 95%. The routine use of supplemental oxygen is not recommended in patients who are not hypoxic (NICE 2008)

Check arterial blood gases if oxygen saturation is less than 95%

Rationale

Accurate monitoring of oxygen saturations with appropriate positioning can minimize the risk of oxygen desaturation (Jones et al. 2007)

In non-hypoxic patients with minor or moderate strokes, supplemental oxygen is considered to be of no clinical benefit and may in fact be detrimental (Potier de la Morandiere and Walter 2003). Further studies are ongoing to clarify this aspect of care

CIRCULATION

Assessment

Pulse 88 beats
per minute

Blood pressure
170/100 mmHg

Management

Monitor and record pulse (rate/rhythm/strength) and BP regularly to detect any change in patient's condition

Record ECG to ensure that the patient is in sinus rhythm

Rationale

Atrial fibrillation is a common cardiac arrhythmia that increases the risk of ischaemic stroke. This will require additional management to prevent the risk of further thromboembolic episodes (Bloe 2011)

(Continued overleaf)

Table 8.1 (*Continued*)

Clinical features	Management and rationale
	In the initial phase of stroke, blood pressure is frequently elevated. However, it is considered that this may represent a physiological response to maintain adequate perfusion of brain tissue
	Immediate treatment to lower BP is not recommended unless this is greater than 200/130 mmHg (NICE 2008) as this may lead to underperfusion of brain tissue
Temperature 37.2°C	*Management*
	Monitor and record temperature regularly
	Guidelines suggest temperature should be maintained within normal limits (ISWP 2008)
	Rationale
	Increased temperature after stroke can be due to disturbances of central temperature regulation, an acute phase response or concurrent infection (Bhalla et al. 2001). Pyrexia in the first 24 hours is associated with greater neurological deficit and dependency in the first three months after stroke Elevated temperature in the first 72 hours is associated with greater mortality (Castillo et al. 2008)
DISABILITY *Assessment*	*Management*
BM 6.2 mmol/L	Monitor and record blood sugar regularly to exclude other conditions which mimic symptoms of acute stroke, e.g. hypoglycaemia
	Hypoglycaemia or hyperglycaemia should be corrected according to local protocols
	ISWP (2008) suggests keeping the blood sugar between 4 mmol/L and 11 mmol/L in the first few days following acute stroke
	Rationale
	Hyperglycaemia in the acute phase of stroke has been shown to have a deleterious effect on neuronal function (Bhalla et al. 2001) and is associated with poorer outcomes
	The Glucose Insulin in Stroke Trial (GIST-UK) stated that both hyper- and hypoglycaemia should be avoided until further evidence is available from ongoing clinical trials (Gray et al. 2007)
Margaret has signs of neurological deficits – right hemiplegia and communication deficits	*Management* Regularly monitor AVPU and Glasgow Coma Scale to assess level of consciousness

It is important to be aware of the limitations of the Glasgow Coma Scale in a patient with aphasia/dysarthria due to a reduced verbal response/cognitive deficits

Support the patient's right side with the use of pillows to maintain correct alignment and position of limbs

Rationale

To establish a baseline for neurological deficits and detect any change in neurological status which may indicate further deterioration in the patient's condition. This may be due to either an evolving ischaemic stroke causing increased cerebral oedema or haemorrhage leading to raised intracranial pressure. Correct positioning is important to prevent any injury which may occur due to sensory inattention or neglect of the affected side and to maintain correct posture and alignment of affected limbs

EXPOSURE
Assessment

Margaret collapsed at home

Management

Head-to-toe examination is required, being mindful to respect the patient's dignity at all times

Rationale

To exclude the presence of any other injuries Margaret may have sustained as a result of her collapse or to detect the presence of incontinence which may be associated with stroke. Urinary incontinence occurs in 40–60% of hospital admissions for stroke in the UK (Barrett 2002). Other urinary problems which may occur include urinary retention and incomplete bladder emptying (Jamieson et al. 2010)

The patient's pressure areas should also be inspected for any redness or signs of developing pressure ulcers due to the patient's immobility or incontinence following the stroke

5 **What additional investigations might Margaret require following admission?**

A Urgent blood samples should be sent for full blood count, urea and electrolytes, cardiac enzymes, serum glucose and coagulation studies as indicated. This will ensure results are available prior to potential administration of thrombolytic therapy and establish baseline parameters to guide ongoing treatment and management.

Neuroimaging is required to distinguish ischaemic from haemorrhagic stroke in the acute stroke patient. Emergency non-contrast computed tomography (CT) of the brain is the initial neuroimaging investigation. This will identify the patient who has suffered a haemorrhage and can identify non-vascular causes of neurological symptoms such as a tumour. However, CT cannot easily identify acute stroke and/or small infarcts and artefact in the brainstem area.

Therefore, magnetic resonance imaging (MRI) is increasingly used as first-line imaging for patients with suspected ischaemic stroke (Chalela et al. 2007). Specialized MRI can identify infarcted areas within a few minutes of onset and therefore allow patients to be identified as suitable candidates for thrombolytic therapy.

> The MRI scan showed no haemorrhage but there was evidence of infarction in the left middle cerebral artery territory. Margaret was therefore considered to be suitable for thrombolytic therapy as she had suffered an ischaemic stroke and was within the three-hour time frame for treatment from the onset of symptoms.

6   **Explain why thrombolytic therapy would be a suitable treatment for Margaret.**

A   The most important aim in acute stroke is restoration of blood flow to the ischaemic area of the brain and surrounding tissue, or penumbra, by breaking up or 'lysing' occlusions in the vascular supply. Prudent use of thrombolytic therapy to promote fibrinolysis and restore blood flow is effective in improving long-term outcomes and reducing disability in patients presenting within three hours of symptom onset (Khaja and Grotta 2007). Following large-scale clinical trials, the thrombolytic drug alteplase has been licensed for use in patients with acute ischaemic stroke who meet the strict criteria set out for administration of the medication. These criteria advise restricting the use of alteplase to patients who are aged 18–80 years, whose symptoms began within the last three hours and who have had intracerebral haemorrhage excluded by brain imaging (see the Think box for further information on exclusion criteria). Local protocols have been developed to assess suitability for treatment which may include additional criteria. Moreover, NICE (2008) recommended that thrombolysis should only be administered in centres with well-developed stroke care facilities to assess and closely monitor these patients. However, additional clinical trials are ongoing to consider the advisability of extending the time frame for the administration of the drug or widening the age group who could potentially benefit from this therapy (Sandercock and members of the International Stroke Trial (IST-3) Collaborative Group 2008). Patients who are alert and do not present with speech impairments can often give reasonably accurate information with respect to the onset of their symptoms. However, this can be more problematic with patients such as Margaret who are dysarthric/aphasic. In these circumstances it may be difficult to accurately establish the time of onset of symptoms, thereby potentially restricting the use of thrombolytic therapy.

> **Think**
>
> Alteplase therapy in patients with acute ischaemic stroke is contraindicated in the following situations because of an increased risk of bleeding, which could result in significant disability or death:
>
> • Evidence of intracranial haemorrhage on pretreatment evaluation.
> • Suspicion of subarachnoid haemorrhage on pretreatment evaluation.

- Recent (within 3 months) intracranial or intraspinal surgery, serious head trauma, or previous stroke.
- History of intracranial haemorrhage.
- Uncontrolled hypertension at time of treatment (e.g. >185 mmHg systolic or >110 mmHg diastolic).
- Seizure at the onset of stroke.
- Active internal bleeding.
- Intracranial neoplasm, arteriovenous malformation, or aneurysm.
- Known bleeding risk factors including but not limited to:
  - Current use of oral anticoagulants (e.g. warfarin sodium) or an international normalized ratio (INR) >1.7 or a prothrombin time (PT) >15 seconds.
- Administration of heparin within 48 hours preceding the onset of stroke and an elevated activated partial thromboplastin time (aPTT) at presentation.
- Platelet count <100,000/mm^3.

(Genentech 2011)

7 **Discuss the issue of consent for administration of thrombolytic therapy in a patient presenting with acute stroke.**

A Informed consent is a widely held principle in nursing and medical practice. The process of obtaining consent informs patients about the treatment and any associated risks, thus respecting patients' autonomy. Written consent is not considered necessary for standard or low risk procedures though in the case of therapeutic interventions with well-recognized risk factors such as thrombolytic therapy, the patients should have the opportunity to make informed decisions about their care and treatment in partnership with health professionals (NICE 2008). However, to obtain consent in the context of acute stroke can be problematic for a number of reasons. First, patients who are facing a sudden critical illness such as a stroke experience considerable shock and distress and may be unable to fully comprehend the implications of the treatment on admission. There is often limited time for patients to become fully cognisant of the implications of the stroke and to understand the risk/benefit ratio of the therapy. Second, the cognitive impairments that accompany stroke can result in communication difficulties or diminished conscious levels which may make the consent process impossible for the patient. Therefore, direct, explicit and autonomous consent from the patient, however ideal, may not always be applicable (Ciccone 2003).

Where appropriate, a family member, e.g. Margaret's husband, should be involved in the discussion to proceed with treatment when the patient is unable to give direct consent. Nevertheless, Greenwood et al. (2009) suggest that Margaret's husband will experience his own shock and anxiety about the prognosis for his wife and uncertainty about what the future may hold and consequently he may also find it difficult to fully grasp the complex information concerning treatment. In these circumstances relatives may not feel able to interpret and represent a patient's wishes. However, decisions to treat must always be taken in the best interests of a patient and where possible consent is obtained from the patient and assent from the next of kin (Fitzpatrick and Birns 2004). Healthcare professionals should follow the Department of Health (2009) guidelines, *Reference Guide to Consent for Examination or Treatment*. Nurses have an important role to play in supporting both patients and relatives at this difficult time by the provision of reassurance, information (both verbal and written) and clear explanation (Innes 2003).

> Despite her communication difficulties Margaret appeared able to convey her wishes through non-verbal expression and gestures and her husband agreed that he felt Margaret would wish to proceed.

8 **Identify the nursing interventions required for a patient receiving thrombolytic therapy following acute stroke.**

A The patient must be admitted to an acute stroke unit or area with staff trained in administration and monitoring for any complications associated with the drug therapy (NICE 2008).

The dose of alteplase (rt-PA) is calculated at a dose of 0.9 mg/kg up to a maximum of 90 mg. 10% of the total dose is given as a bolus over 1 minute with the remaining 90% infused intravenously over 1 hour (Genentech 2011).

Table 8.2 gives the nursing interventions required when administering thrombolytic therapy after a stroke.

Table 8.2 Nursing interventions when administering thrombolytic therapy

Nursing interventions	Rationale
Weigh the patient or estimate weight as accurately as possible	To facilitate accurate calculation of drug dosage
Place patient on cardiac monitor prior to commencement of treatment	To enable detection of potential derangement in cardiac function such as atrial fibrillation or other arrhythmias
Record temperature, pulse, blood pressure, oxygen saturation and neurological status prior to therapy, then every 15 minutes for 2 hours, every 30 minutes for the next 6 hours, hourly for the next 6 hours and 4-hourly if condition is stable (Rowat et al. 2009)	To detect signs of haemorrhage or deterioration in the patient's condition during or post-treatment due to reperfusion of the affected area in the brain tissue
The use of a manual sphygmomanometer is recommended during therapy and in the 24 hours following treatment Report any signs of bleeding or bruising immediately	It is suggested by Innes and the International Stroke Trial (IST-3) Nurse Collaborative Group (2003) that automated machines that use high inflation pressures should be avoided during treatment. Frequent use of mechanical cuffs can cause severe bruising or bleeding

Report any changes in vital signs or neurological observations promptly to medical staff

The foremost concern with respect to treatment with thrombolytic agents is haemorrhagic transformation which should be suspected if the patient demonstrates increased drowsiness, headache or neurological deterioration (Khaja and Grotta 2007)

Avoid central venous access, arterial punctures and injections for the first 24 hours and exercise care in removing indwelling intravenous catheters Antiplatelets, anticoagulants and non-steroidal anti-inflammatory drugs (NSAIDs) should be withheld for 24 hours after the bolus of thrombolysis is given (Khaja and Grotta 2007)

Invasive procedures such as urinary catheterization and nasogastric tube insertion should be avoided where possible to prevent trauma which may result in excessive bleeding Guidelines recommend that aspirin is delayed for 24 hours following thrombolysis to minimize the risk of haemorrhage (ISWP 2008)

Maintain the patient on bedrest for 24 hours following administration of the drug

To facilitate rigorous patient monitoring with particular attention to patient safety if patient has sensory inattention or neglect

Arrange repeat CT/MRI scan in 24 hours

To evaluate the effect of treatment

Margaret made good progress following thrombolysis treatment although some deficits remained in her speech. However, she became independent in activities of living again reasonable quickly and was able to return home on an early discharge programme with input from the community stroke team. She will also attend the community speech and language therapy service for further treatment.

Key points
- Time is of the essence in acute stroke.
- Thrombolysis is an important emergent treatment for acute ischaemic stroke although there are well-recognized risks associated with this treatment.
- Early recognition and treatment are vital to reduce long-term disability.

REFERENCES

Barrett, J.A. (2002) Bladder and bowel problems after a stroke, *Reviews in Clinical Gerontology*, 12(3): 253–67.

Bath, P.M.W. and Lees, K.R. (2000) ABC of arterial and venous disease: acute stroke, *British Medical Journal*, 320: 900–23.

Bhalla, A., Wolfe, C.D.A. and Rudd, A.G. (2001) Management of acute physiological parameters after stroke, *QJM: Monthly Journal of the Association of Physicians*, 94(3): 167–72.

Bloe, C. (2011) Atrial fibrillation and primary stroke prevention, *Nursing Standard*, 26(6): 49–57.

Borthwick, S. (2012) Communication impairment in patients following stroke. *Nursing Standard*, 26(19): 35–41.

Castillo, J., Davalos, A., Marrugat, J. and Noya, M. (2008) Timing for fever related brain damage in acute ischaemic stroke, *Stroke*, 29(12): 2455–60.

Chalela, J.A., Kidwell, C.S., Nentwich, I.M. et al. (2007) Magnetic resonance imaging and computed tomography in the emergency assessment of patients with suspected acute stroke: a prospective comparison, *The Lancet*, 369: 293–8.

Ciccone, A. (2003) Consent to thrombolysis in acute ischaemic stroke: from trial to practice. *The Lancet Neurology*, 2(6): 375–8.

Department of Health (2009) *Reference Guide to Consent for Examination or Treatment*, 2nd edn. London: Department of Health.

Fitzpatrick, M. and Birns, J. (2004) Thrombolysis for acute stroke and the role of the nurse, *British Journal of Nursing*, 13(20): 1170–4.

Genentech (2011) *Alteplase Prescribing Information*. San Francisco: Genentech.

Gray, C.S., Hildreth, A.J., Sandercock, P.A. et al. (2007) Glucose-potassium-insulin infusions in the management of post-stroke hyperglycaemia: the UK Glucose Insulin in Stroke Trial (GIST-UK), *The Lancet Neurology*, 6(5): 397–406.

Greenwood, N., Mackenzie, A., Wilson, N. and Cloud, G. (2009) Managing uncertainty in life after stroke: a qualitative study of the experiences of established and new informal carers in the first 3 months after discharge. *International Journal of Nursing Studies*, 46(8): 1122–33.

Harbinson, J., Hossain, O., Jenkinson, D. et al. (2003) Diagnostic accuracy of stroke referrals from primary care, emergency room physicians and ambulance staff using the face arm speech test, *Stroke*, 34(1): 71–6.

Hinkle, J.L., Manoj, A., Brook, S., Webb, A., Muangpaisan, W., Kennedy, J. and Buchan, A.M. (2007) Nursing triage of patients with acute stroke, *Nursing Times*, 103(31): 32–3.

Innes, K. and International Stroke Trial (IST-3) Stroke Nurse Collaborative Group (2003) Thrombolysis for acute ischaemic stroke: core nursing requirements, *British Journal of Nursing*, 12: 416–24.

ISWP (Intercollegiate Stroke Working Party) (2008) *National Clinical Guidelines for Stroke*, 3rd edn. London: Royal College of Physicians.

Jamieson, K. et al. (2010) Urinary dysfunction: assessment and management in stroke patients, *Nursing Standard*, 25(3): 49–55.

Jones, S.P., Leathley, M.J., McAdam, J.J. and Watkins, C.L. (2007) Physiological monitoring in acute stroke: a literature review, *Journal of Advanced Nursing*, 60(6): 577–94.

Kelly, T. et al. (2010) Review of the evidence to support oral hygiene in stroke patients, *Nursing Standard*, 24(37): 35–8.

Khaja, A.M. and Grotta, J.C. (2007) Established treatments for acute ischaemic stroke, *The Lancet*, 369: 319–30.

Lawson, C. and Gibbons, D. (2009) Acute stroke management in emergency departments, *Emergency Nurse*, 17(5): 30–4.

McCance, K.L. and Huether, S.E. (2006) *Pathophysiology: The Biologic Basis for Disease in Adults and Children*, 5th edn. St Louis, MO: Elsevier Mosby.

NICE (National Institute for Health and Clinical Excellence) (2008) *Stroke Diagnosis and Initial Management of Acute Stroke and Transient Ischaemic Attack (TIA)*. London: NICE.

Nor, A., Davis, J., Sen, B., Shipsey, D., Louw, S.J., Dyker, A.G., Davis, M. and Ford, G.A. (2005) The Recognition of Stroke in the Emergency Room (ROSIER) scale: development and validation of a stroke recognition instrument, *The Lancet Neurology*, 4(1): 727–34.

Potier de la Morandiere, K. and Walter, D. (2003) Oxygen therapy in acute stroke, *Emergency Medicine Journal*, 20: 547–53.

Rowat, A. et al. (2009) Using the mnemonic 'brain attack' in the management of acute stroke, *Nursing Standard*, 24(6): 50–7.

Sandercock, P. and members of the IST-3 Collaborative Group (2008) The third International Stroke Trial (IST-3) of thrombolysis for acute ischaemic stroke, *Trials*, 9: 37.

Soames, J. and Bergman, D.L., (2007) ABCD's of acute stroke intervention, *Journal of Emergency Nursing*, 33(3): 228–34.

Status epilepticus
Karen Page

Case outline

Tom Patterson, a 24-year-old university student was admitted to the A&E unit via ambulance mid-morning. He was recently diagnosed as having epilepsy, though he has been well controlled and seizure-free for generalized tonic-clonic seizures for the past 3 months on his current medication of carbamazepine 200 mg orally T.I.D. However, this morning he experienced a seizure without recovering consciousness during a written examination and the invigilator called the emergency services. On attending the scene the paramedic witnessed Tom experience a second tonic-clonic seizure and there-fore a stat dose of buccal midazolam 10 mg was administered by the paramedic prior to transporting the patient to the A&E unit.

---

1 **Describe the clinical features which characterize a tonic-clonic seizure.**

A Tonic-clonic seizures are often referred to as generalized seizures and usually have several stages:

1 *Premonitory phase*: Some patients may experience a warning sign that a seizure is imminent.
2 *Tonic phase*: During the tonic phase the person goes stiff as the muscles contract. If the person is standing, he or she will fall to the ground. The person may appear to cry out as the muscles in the lungs contract and force air out through the vocal cords. Their breathing becomes irregular, or the person may experience a period of apnoea, resulting in a lack of oxygen in the lungs causing cyanosis. Occasionally the patient may bite their tongue or become incontinent.
3 *Clonic phase*: During the clonic phase the stiffness passes to give way to intermittent contraction and relaxation of muscles that produce rhythmical powerful jerking movements of the face, body and limbs. Hyperventilation, tachycardia, sweating and excessive production of saliva may accompany this. This can last for some minutes before the person enters the final phase.
4 *Post-ictal phase*: The muscles relax and person goes limp. They will have a depressed conscious level. Slowly, normal colour returns and consciousness gradually returns to normal. They may be groggy and confused and may not be able to remember the seizure.

Recovery time varies from minutes to hours. Many people complain of a headache and aching limbs which can last for some time after the seizure.

(Epilepsy Action 2011)

2   **Explain the physiological changes associated with an epileptic seizure.**

A   The nervous system is a complex highly organized network of neurones. Neurones have the property of electrical excitability and function by generating and transmitting action potentials (small electrical signals) in response to stimuli. These action potentials or impulses are then passed from neurone to neurone via neurotransmitters across neuronal synapses. Both excitatory (aspartate and glutamate) and inhibitory neurotransmitters (gamma aminobutyric acid (GABA)) are present in the central nervous system. Spread of electrical activity between neurones is normally limited and synchronous discharge of neurones takes place in restricted groups, producing the normal neuronal communication seen on EEG recordings. During a seizure, large groups of neurones are repetitively and synchronously activated while inhibitory synaptic activity between neurones fails. This produces the high voltage spike and wave activity which is the hallmark of epilepsy (Kumar and Clark 2005). A seizure is the physical manifestation of this abnormal electrical activity although it is not exclusively caused by epilepsy. Other conditions such as diabetes, migraine, syncope, and cardiovascular conditions can cause seizure or seizure-like symptoms (Welsh and Kerley 2009).

3   **Define status epilepticus (SE) and explain the requirement to treat this as a medical emergency.**

A   SE represents a failure of innate cellular mechanisms to prevent sustained seizure activity and is associated with high morbidity and mortality if not treated promptly (NICE 2012). Traditionally generalized convulsive status epilepticus was defined as a condition in which there was 30 minutes or more of continuous seizure activity or a series of seizures without return to full consciousness between seizures. Prolonged seizure activity may also evolve into more subtle neurological findings such as ocular deviation, fine nystagmus, or subtle jaw, finger or eyelid twitching before progressing to only electrical activity without visible physical correlation (Manno 2003). The major physiological changes that occur in SE are related to the greatly increased cerebral blood flow and metabolism, massive autonomic nervous system activity and cardiovascular changes. In phase 1, although cerebral metabolism is increased by seizure activity compensatory physiological mechanisms protect cerebral tissue from metabolic damage or hypoxia. In phase 2, these compensatory mechanisms break down and there is an increasing risk of cerebral damage. Cerebral metabolic demands become unsustainable, resulting in cerebral hypoxia and raised intracranial pressure (ICP). Systemic changes include hyperpyrexia, hypoglycaemia, acidosis, falling blood pressure, reduced cardiac output and respiratory impairment. In addition to these changes, there is also a direct toxic effect on neurones associated with the seizure. This results in calcium influx into neurones and a cascade of events resulting in necrosis and apoptosis or death of neurones (Shorvon 2001; Hayes 2004). The focus of SE treatment is therefore early seizure termination to prevent cerebral damage. Moreover, treatment of the early stages of status epilepticus is likely to be more successful then treatment in the later stages as time-dependent development of resistance to anti-epileptic drugs (AEDs) has been observed (Chen and Wasterlain 2006). Consequently it is recommended that treatment should commence as soon as it is apparent that the seizure activity is persisting (continuous or intermittent seizures lasting more than 5 minutes without full recovery of consciousness between seizures) or there is a significant worsening in the patient's condition (Walker and Shorvon 2009).

4 **Explain why the paramedic administered buccal midazolam to Tom prior to admission to hospital.**

A As it is essential to terminate seizure activity the paramedic was following the training and management guidelines developed by the Joint Epilepsy Council (JEC 2005) for the administration of benzodiazepines. The benzodiazepines including diazepam, lorazepam and midazolam are the preferred initial choice for treatment of status epilepticus, mainly because of their rapid onset of action, and effectiveness in aborting seizures. Their primary pharmacological actions are thought to be related to a benzodiazepine receptor-mediated enhancement or facilitation of GABA transmission, which is the main inhibitory neurotransmitter at central nervous system synapses. Stimulation of this receptor leads to inhibition of neural transmission by decreasing the cells' ability to initiate an action potential, thereby reducing seizure activity (Manno 2003).

Traditionally treatment has involved administration of rectal diazepam to patients who are experiencing tonic-clonic seizures prior to admission to achieve rapid seizure control. However, buccal midazolam is emerging as initial therapy for patients in the community (JEC 2005). Buccal preparations are medicines administered into the buccal space, which is between the inside of the cheek and gum in the mouth. Since it can be given via the buccal route it does not carry the difficulties of administration associated with rectal diazepam and furthermore is more socially acceptable and dignified for patients (Queally 2007). Midazolam is a highly lipid soluble drug which allows rapid absorption and cerebral penetration to achieve sufficient therapeutic serum levels to suppress seizure activity. However, it has an extremely short duration of action which can lead to a high reoccurrence rate of seizures and consequently the patient should be transferred immediately to hospital for further observation (McKenry et al. 2006).

5 **As you are admitting Tom, he experiences another seizure. What is the immediate nursing care required at this point?**

A From a nursing perspective, the priorities are maintaining patient safety and airway management.

Check points: nursing priorities

Ensuring a safe environment

- Make a note of the time the seizure commenced and call for assistance.
- Do not attempt to restrain patient movement. Muscular contractions are strong and restraint can lead to injury and should therefore be avoided.
- If the patient is in bed or on a trolley, remove the pillows and raise the side rails.
- Use padding to protect the patient from injury particularly head injury or injuries to the limbs.
- Ensure a safe environment during any seizure activity by moving any objects which are likely to cause harm out of the way.
- Stay with the patient and screen the patient from other people so protecting his or her privacy and dignity, particularly if the patient has been incontinent.

- Provide emotional support and orientation as the patient begins to recover from the seizure and continue to observe until fully recovered.

Airway management

During a seizure the patient may experience a period of apnoea and become cyanosed; however, this is generally brief and should not create a problem unless the airway is blocked.

- Airway management assists with maintaining adequate cerebral oxygenation; however, *Do not attempt to place anything in the patient's mouth during a seizure.* Any injury to the tongue is likely to have already occurred and such action may result in further damage to the gums and teeth or indeed the nurse's fingers!
- As soon as possible, place the patient in the recovery position with the head flexed forward, loosening any restrictive clothing. Positioning the patient in the left lateral position will decrease the risk of aspiration as it allows the tongue to fall forward and facilitates drainage of saliva and mucus. This assists in maintaining adequate cerebral oxygenation and protects against aspiration; however, this may not be possible until the seizure activity has stopped.
- Administer oxygen as prescribed to maintain SpO_2 levels >94% as hypoxia is often severe during a seizure.
- Wipe away any excessive salivary secretions. Use suction as necessary to clear secretions.
- Do not give the person anything to eat or drink until they are fully recovered.
- Report and document the duration and features of the seizure (Hayes 2004; Whittaker 2004).

6 **Tom remains very drowsy following the seizure. Describe the ongoing assessment and monitoring of the patient.**

A Follow the ABCDE procedure as shown in Table 9.1.

Table 9.1 The ABCDE procedure in the case of epileptic seizures

ABCDE	Nursing intervention
A = Airway	Seizures and the medications used to control them can impair the level of consciousness and airway patency, so continue to monitor airway. A spontaneously maintained airway may still be at risk from aspiration in SE due to the excess salivation which occurred during the seizure. Suction may be required to remove excess secretions. Airway patency can be secured by means of a nasopharyngeal airway in patients with tightly clenched teeth or when the patient has an active gag reflex. Oxygen should be administered as prescribed to maintain oxygen saturations >94% (Walker 2005). If there is respiratory compromise or if seizures persist, prepare to assist with intubation to maintain the airway

B = Breathing   Record and monitor respiratory rate, pulse oximetry and arterial blood gas (if seizure activity is prolonged) to measure the extent of acidosis present and respiratory function (SIGN 2003). Assess breathing; observe for laboured breathing or added sounds to determine the presence or extent of any ventilatory difficulties

C = Circulation   Record and monitor pulse, blood pressure, ECG and temperature. Initiate cardiac monitoring. Obtain IV access, if not already present, for fluid replacement and drug administration, preferably with 0.9% sodium chloride rather than dextrose solutions as precipitation may occur with the use of some AEDs such as phenytoin. AEDs should not be mixed so if more than one drug is required, two separate IV lines should be inserted. Wide-bore cannula should be used as many AEDs cause phlebitis and thrombosis at the site of infusion (Walker and Shorvon 2009). Obtain blood specimens for the following investigations: blood sugar, full blood picture including platelets and clotting factors, urea and electrolytes, renal and liver function tests, AED levels and a toxicology screen. A urinary catheter may be required to monitor urinary output if hypotension is present or patient remains unconscious

D = Disability   Record and monitor neurological observations. AVPU and the Glasgow Coma Scale should be recorded to establish level of consciousness or identify signs of neurological deficit. Obtain capillary blood sugar level to exclude hypoglycaemia. Assess pain scale if possible

E = Exposure   Check for signs of injury, particularly head injury, or evidence of any other abnormalities such as rash or bruising

---

The ABCDE assessment reveals the following information:

Blood pressure: 180/100 mmHg
Pulse: 120 beats per minute
Respirations: 24 breaths/minute
SpO$_2$: 96% with oxygen therapy
Temperature: 38.4°C
Cardiac monitor indicates sinus rhythm.
Blood glucose is within normal limits, ruling out hypoglycaemia as an easily correctible cause of Tom's seizures.
ABG results indicate adequate oxygenation; however, metabolic acidosis is apparent. This is often present in generalized status epilepticus and reflects sustained muscular activity. This is self-correcting once seizures are controlled and rarely requires treatment (Manno 2003).

7   Discuss the AEDs commonly used for the patient with continuing seizure activity and identify the related nursing implications.

A   • *Lorazepam* can be used in the early stages of status epilepticus following an initial dose of a benzodiazepine, such as diazepam or midazolam. Lorazepam is preferable to these drugs because of its lack of accumulation in lipid stores, strong cerebral binding and long duration of action (about 12 hours) leading to a smaller chance of reoccurrence of seizures. Lorazepam shares the side effects of all the benzodiazepine drugs used in SE; however, sudden hypotension or respiratory collapse is less likely.

- *Phenytoin* is a barbiturate-like drug that is ideally suited for rapid control of seizures with the advantage of a long duration of action. Phenytoin blocks voltage-sensitive sodium channels, thus stabilizing neuronal membranes at the cell body, axon and synapse and so inhibiting repetitive neuronal firing, limiting the spread of neuronal or seizure activity. Phenytoin causes relatively little respiratory or cerebral depression although hypotension can occur.
- *Fosphenytoin* which is administered as an inactive form (or prodrug) was introduced to overcome the problems associated with phenytoin. It is rapidly converted to an active form in the body and has the same pharmacological effect as phenytoin. Although it is considerably more expensive, this drug causes less phlebitis, reduced cardiovascular adverse effects, is easier to administer and better tolerated by patients. The usual dose is based on phenytoin equivalents; however, medical errors have resulted from dosing errors related to this product so extra care is required when calculating drug dosages (McKenry et al. 2006).
- *Phenobarbital* is a barbiturate that prevents seizure activity by increasing GABA-mediated cellular inhibition in a similar manner to benzodiazepines. Although phenobarbital has been used for many years to control SE, it is now considered to be a third-line drug to treat SE because of its serious side effect profile. It profoundly depresses respirations and consciousness levels and can cause severe hypotension secondary to peripheral vasodilation and decreased cardiac contractility.

Table 9.2 shows the effects and nursing implications of different drugs in the case of epileptic seizures.

Table 9.2 Effects of different drugs and implications in the case of an epileptic seizure

Status	Drug	Nursing implications
Early status 0–30 minutes	Lorazepam 0.1 mg/kg. Usually given as a 4 mg bolus repeated once after 10–20 minutes	Monitor for hypotension, tachycardia and respiratory depression
Established status 30–60/90 minutes	Phenytoin 18–20 mg/kg in non-glucose containing solutions at a maximum rate of 50 mg/min. (Walker and Shorvon 2009). Older patients, debilitated patients or those with renal impairment will require a lower dose and a slower rate of administration Or Fosphenytoin infusion at a dose of 15–20 mg Phenytoin equivalent (PE)/kg at a rate of 150 mg PE/min.	IV phenytoin is very irritating to the vein. Monitor for signs of phlebitis Monitor BP to detect hypotension ECG monitoring is mandatory during administration of both phenytoin and fosphenytoin to detect possible cardiac arrthymias Extra care is required to minimize drug errors when using fosphenytoin (McKenry et al. 2006)

	And/Or Phenobarbitone bolus of 10 mg/kg at a rate of 100 mg/minute	Monitor respirations, conscious level and BP Transfer to ICU is required with intubation and intensive monitoring
Refractory status after 60–90 minutes	Full anaesthesia is required with either propofol, midazolam or thiopentone. Anaesthesia should be continued for 12–24 hours after the last clinical or EEG noted seizure then gradually tapered off	EEG monitoring should be initiated as the anaesthesia will mask the motor symptoms of epilepsy

Source: NICE (2012); Walker and Shorvon (2009); BNF (2011).

Tom was given a stat. dose of lorazepam 4 mg following his seizure on arrival in A&E. Subsequently he had one further seizure before the seizure activity terminated and he slowly began to recover consciousness although he remained very drowsy. Paracetamol 1g rectally was administered to control his pyrexia and he was admitted to the neurology ward for continued observations. Blood results indicated evidence of leucocytosis with a carbamazepine level of 5 mcg/mL.

8   **Identify the possible causes of Tom's seizure activity.**

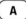   In patients with an established diagnosis of epilepsy, SE can be precipitated by drug withdrawal or failure to take the prescribed drugs, intercurrent illness or metabolic disturbance. It is also important for the nurse to check for any possible triggers such as illness, sleep deprivation, use of alcohol or recreational drug use, stress or hormonal changes in women including menstruation (Epilepsy Action 2012). Tom acknowledged that he had been unwell with flu-like symptoms in the past week. He had also been rather stressed and studying late into the night to prepare for his end-of-year examinations. Sleep deprivation has been shown to alter cerebral electrical activity, therefore repeatedly staying up late may precipitate a seizure in some patients (Epilepsy Action 2010). As with all medications, non-compliance must be considered when therapeutic regimes become ineffective. Tom stated that he had continued to take his medication; however, as levels were sub-therapeutic (carbamazepine normal range 6–12 mcg/mL) on admission, this was reviewed by the consultant. Compliance with medication is crucial as a missed dose may result in a seizure a few days later and taking an extra dose will not prevent an impending seizure (McKenry et al. 2006). Having ruled out missed doses of medication, sub-therapeutic levels of the drug are characteristic of carbamazepine to induce hepatic cytochrome P450 enzymes and so stimulate its own metabolism. This can significantly decrease the drug's half-life and will necessitate an increase in dosage for the drug to be effective (McKenry et al. 2006). Tom's prescription was therefore increased to 400 mg slow release tablets B.D.

> **Key points**
> - SE is a neurological emergency.
> - Prompt attention should be paid to Airway, Breathing and Circulation (ABC).
> - First-line treatment should be with benzodiazepines; however, continued monitoring is essential to detect complications associated with AEDs.

REFERENCES

BNF (British National Formulary) (2011) *BNF 62*. London: September BMJ Group and Pharmaceutical Press.

Chen, J.W.Y. and Wasterlain, C.G. (2006) Status epilepticus: pathophysiology and management in adults, *The Lancet Neurology*, 5: 246–56.

Epilepsy Action (2010) *Sleep and Epilepsy*. Available at: www.epilepsyaction.org.uk (accessed 18 January 2012).

Epilepsy Action (2011) *Tonic-clonic Seizures*. Available at: www.epilepsyaction.org.uk (accessed 18 January 2012).

Epilepsy Action (2012) *Seizure Triggers*. Available at: www.epilepsyaction.org.uk (accessed 18 January 2012).

Hayes, C. (2004) Clinical skills: practical guide for managing adults with epilepsy, *British Journal of Nursing*, 13(7): 380–7.

JEC (Joint Epilepsy Council) (2005) *A Guideline on Training Standards for the Administration of Buccal Midazolam*. Leeds: JEC.

Kumar, P. and Clark, M. (2005) *Clinical Medicine*, 6th edn. London: Elsevier Saunders.

Manno, E.M. (2003) New management strategies in the treatment of status epilepticus, *Mayo Clinic Procedures*, 78: 505–18.

McKenry, L., Tessier, E. and Hogan, M. (2006) *Mosby's Pharmacology in Nursing*, 22nd edn. St Louis, MO: Elsevier Mosby.

NICE (National Institute for Health and Clinical Excellence) (2012) *The Epilepsies: The Diagnosis and Management of the Epilepsies in Adults and Children in Primary and Secondary Care*. London: NICE.

Queally, C. (2007) The use of buccal midazolam in emergency seizure management in epilepsy, *British Journal of Neuroscience Nursing*, 3(6): 272–5.

Shorvon, S. (2001) The management of status epilepticus, *Journal of Neurology, Neurosurgery and Psychiatry*, 70(Suppl. ii): 22–7.

SIGN (Scottish Intercollegiate Guidelines Network) (2003) *Diagnosis and Management of Epilepsy in Adults*. Edinburgh: Scottish Intercollegiate Guidelines Network.

Walker, M. (2005) Status epilepticus: an evidence-based guide, *British Medical Journal*, 331(7518): 673.

Walker, M.C. and Shorvon, S.D. (2009) Treatment of tonic-clonic status epilepticus, in J.W. Sander, M.C. Walker, and J.E. Smalls (eds) *Epilepsy from Benchside to Bedside: A Practical Guide to Epilepsy*, 12th edn. Chalfont St Giles: International League against Epilepsy and The National Society for Epilepsy.

Welsh, R. and Kerley, S. (2009) Nursing patients with epilepsy in secondary care settings, *Nursing Standard*, 23(36): 49–56.

Whittaker, N. (2004) *Disorders and Interventions*. Basingstoke: Palgrave Macmillan.

PART 5
Digestive System

Acute abdomen

Aidín McKinney

Case outline

Mr Sam Smith is a 62-year-old man who has been admitted to A&E with a four-day history of colicky abdominal pain. He has been feeling nauseated and has vomited on a few occasions this morning. His lips look very dry and he has difficulty talking as his mouth is so dry. He has also complained that his bowels have not moved for at least four days and his abdomen appears to be a bit distended. He is quite anxious about his condition. On questioning, he estimates his pain score to be 8 out of 10.

His vital signs are:

Temperature: 37.4°C
Pulse: 110 beats per minute
Respiratory rate (RR): 25 breaths per minute
BP: 125/80 mmHg.

---

1 **Discuss how Sam should be assessed, using the ABCDE approach.**

A Abdominal pain is one of the most common reasons that people may seek medical attention. However, it can be challenging to identify the specific cause of the abdominal pain because of the diversity of symptoms that the patient may present with. Obtaining an accurate history and carrying out a structured and systematic assessment of the patient are therefore vital to aid a timely diagnosis and to differentiate between abdominal pain caused by acute or non-acute conditions (Cole et al. 2006).

PAST MEDICAL HISTORY

When a patient presents with abdominal pain, there are some key factors that need to be considered which may provide significant clues as to why they are experiencing this pain. Some of these factors include enquiring as to whether the patient has had previous surgery. This may indicate a recurrence of the previous problem, adhesions or post-operative infection. Also obtain a medication history – a patient taking multiple medications is at increased risk of damage to the liver, and patients taking NSAIDs are at increased risk of gastric irritation/bleeding. It is also worth considering whether the patient has a history of conditions such as

Crohn's disease or peptic ulcer disease. Finally, in females, it is important to consider pregnancy as acute abdominal pain in early pregnancy may be indicative of an ectopic pregnancy (Cole et al. 2006).

When a patient presents with an acute illness, it is important to carry out a quick, structured and prioritized method of assessment. It is now well recognized that the ABCDE approach to assessment is probably the clearest and most commonly used approach to use when assessing the acutely ill patient (Ahern and Philpot 2002). Table 10.1 presents the ABCDE procedure for checking Sam's condition.

Table 10.1 The ABCDE procedure in the case of an acute abdomen

ABCDE	Nursing intervention
A = Airway	Assess whether the airway is patent. A simple question such as 'How are you?' establishes two things – the patient's level of consciousness and whether the airway is patent (Ahern and Philpot 2002). It is evident that Sam's airway is patent as he is speaking to us. However, as he is vomiting, it is important to recognize that this has the potential to obstruct the airway and therefore needs to be monitored closely
B = Breathing	Assess the rate, depth and ease of respiration. The normal rate is around 12–18 breaths per minute. This is important to be aware of as respiratory rate deviation from normal is now widely accepted as being one of the earliest indicators of patient deterioration. As Sam's respiratory rate is 25 breaths per minute, it is evident that his condition has deteriorated and he is acutely unwell. It is also important at this stage to listen to the chest and to observe the accessory muscles for any other signs of increased respiratory effort or difficulty breathing such as reduced oxygen saturation levels
C = Circulation	When assessing circulation, it is important to consider heart rate and blood pressure, look at the skin for signs of reduced peripheral perfusion, determine capillary refill time and observe for any signs of haemorrhage, fluid loss or for signs of internal bleeding. Cardiac monitoring should also be used when available (Ahern and Philpot 2002). In Sam's case, it is evident that his heart rate has increased. Blood pressure is still within normal limits; however, it is important to be aware that hypotension is a late sign of shock and thus his blood pressure may be within normal limits at present due to the compensatory mechanisms that exist within the body to maintain homeostasis. It is important therefore to monitor this closely as it may deteriorate if or when the compensatory mechanisms become exhausted. It may also be useful to monitor the patient's temperature at this point as it is evident that his temperature is slightly elevated at 37.4°C

D = Disability

This refers to the assessment of consciousness level. A quick, easy scoring system that can be used is the AVPU score which assesses whether the patient is alert, can respond to voice, pain or is unresponsive (Ahern and Philpot 2002). It is apparent that Sam is alert and therefore does not require any further assessment under this area for now. However, depending on the patient's illness or signs of altering levels of consciousness, it may also be useful to assess using the Glasgow Coma Scale. Monitoring blood sugars for signs of hypo-or hyperglycaemia can also be useful to explain altered levels of consciousness

E = Exposure

This is a top-to-toe, front-to-back examination of the patient observing for any obvious signs of bleeding, bruising, swelling, rashes or signs of previous surgery. At this stage it is also important to assess the patient's level of pain if you have not done so already (Ahern and Philpot 2002). On examination, it is obvious that Sam has a distended abdomen, is complaining of colicky abdominal pain and is scoring his pain as 8 out of 10

2 **Identify Sam's main problems and explain these in relation to the underlying pathophysiology.**

A Sam's main problems are:

Colicky abdominal pain
Nausea and vomiting
No bowel movements
Temperature 37.4°C
Pulse 110 beats per minute
Respiratory rate 25 breaths per minute
Dry mouth
Anxiety
Distended abdomen

Table 10.2 overleaf shows his main problems and their pathophysiology.

3 **On assessment, Sam indicates his pain is at level 8 on a 0–10 pain tool. Discuss what type of pain relief you should administer and why.**

A As the pain is described as being quite severe in nature, the drug of choice is likely to be opioid analgesics. Quite often morphine or pethidine are common opioid preparations that are indicated for moderate to severe pain (Hughes 2005). It has been noted, however, that some surgeons can be reluctant to use analgesia in case it may mask clinical findings and therefore delay diagnosis. However, a Cochrane Review conducted by Manterola et al. (2011) evaluated clinical trials comparing administration of opioid analgesia to no analgesia in patients with acute abdominal pain. They concluded that opioid analgesics were helpful in terms of patient comfort and do not mask clinical findings or delay diagnosis.

Table 10.2 Sam's main problems and their pathophysiology

Patient problem	Pathophysiology
Colicky abdominal pain	Colicky abdominal pain often occurs in the case of small bowel obstruction. Pain is often felt around the umbilical or epigastric areas of the abdomen. This occurs because the natural peristaltic action of the gut is attempting to push the fluid levels that are rising past the obstruction. However, if the large bowel is obstructed, it is more likely that the middle and lower abdomen will be affected, and the pain is likely to be more cramp-like in nature and is generally described as being of a more gradual onset (Hughes 2005). However, if strangulation of the bowel occurs, the pain will lose its colicky character and become more constant and severe as ischaemia progresses to necrosis or perforation (Mattson Porth 2007)
Nausea and vomiting	Fluids will accumulate from impaired water and electrolyte absorption. There will also be increased secretions from the bowel wall with net movement of fluid from the vascular space to the intestinal lumen. Gas from swallowed air and to a lesser extent from bacterial overgrowth will further contribute to the distended bowel and this will further decrease the bowel's ability to absorb water. Within 24 hrs, up to 8 litres of fluid and electrolytes can accumulate in the lumen. Fluid will therefore be passed back or backflow to the stomach, causing vomiting (Mattson Porth 2007) If the obstruction is high, the tendency for vomiting is particularly raised, and usually causes more severe vomiting (Baines 1997). Higher fluid levels will be associated with the small bowel as the majority of the fluid is absorbed after it passes through the ileo-caecal valve. If the obstruction is lower, vomiting may not occur until later and this may contain faecal matter (Hughes 2005). Vomiting will also lead to decreased plasma levels in the blood. This will increase the red blood concentration, elevating haematocrit levels and will therefore increase the patient's risk of developing thrombi. Alterations in the patient's electrolytes may also occur, resulting in a significant loss of hydrogen and potassium ions, leading to a metabolic acidosis (Smeltzer et al. 2008)
No bowel movements	Some patients may find that they become constipated. Bowel contents, stools or flatus may be unable to move past the obstruction. In small bowel obstruction, this may be due to hernias, adhesions, tumours or Crohn's disease (Longmore et al. 2004). In large bowel obstruction, this may be due to carcinoma, diverticulitis or inflammatory bowel disease
Raised temperature	A raised temperature will suggest an inflammatory response or the presence of a bacterial infection especially if peritonitis develops (Cole et al. 2006)

Tachycardia	Tachycardia can be linked to the compensatory mechanism associated with hypovolaemia as the heart attempts to circulate the lowered blood volume due to the fluid shifts that have occurred (Mattson Porth 2007)
Respiratory rate 25 breaths per minute	The respiratory rate is increased as the heart and lungs work together to oxygenate the small volume of circulating blood and remove excess carbon dioxide from the blood. Increased respiratory rate is an early indicator of deterioration in the acutely unwell patient (Ahern and Philpot 2002)
Dry mouth	The vomiting will prevent reabsorption which will ultimately lead to severe fluid and electrolyte disturbances. Extracellular fluid volume and plasma volume will decrease leading to dehydration, resulting in a dry mouth and lips (Hughes 2005)
Anxiety	The patient is likely to be very anxious due to the pain, nausea and vomiting. Stimulation of the sympathetic nervous system (SNS) and the subsequent release of adrenaline will further contribute to the anxiety
Distended abdomen	Due to the obstruction, fluids accumulate in the area. If untreated, the distension resulting from bowel obstruction tends to perpetuate itself by causing atony of the bowel and leads to further distension. Distension will also be further aggravated by the accumulation of gases, the majority of which will be derived from swallowed air. As the process continues, the distension moves upwards towards the mouth, involving additional segments of bowel. This increased pressure in the intestine may compromise mucosal blood flow and ultimately may result in strangulation or interruption of blood flow to the bowel. This can cause necrosis, gangrenous changes and ultimately, perforation of the bowel (Mattson Porth 2007)

4 **Discuss the management and administration of opioid analgesics and Sam's after-care post-administration of this drug.**

A Assess pain thoroughly before and after administration, assessing for the location of the pain, the type, intensity, severity and duration. Administer the drug safely following the policy and guidelines within the *Standards for Medicines Management* (NMC 2010).

Check points: drug administration

Monitor for side effects, including:

- *Cardiovascular effects*: hypotension, palpitations and flushing.
- *Central nervous system effects*: sedation, disorientation, euphoria, light-headedness, addiction, pupillary constriction.

- *Respiratory effects*: respiratory depression, bronchospasm, aggravation of cough suppression.
- *Gastrointestinal effects*: nausea, vomiting, reduction in peristalsis, constipation.
- *Urinary tract effects:* urinary retention.
- *Educate* the patient on some of these and monitor for any side effects.

Monitoring may include:

- Monitoring respiratory rate and oxygen saturation levels.
- Monitoring blood pressure.
- Monitoring urinary output.
- Monitoring for nausea/vomiting.
- Ensure opioid antagonist (naloxone) is available in case of respiratory depression.
- Other effects to monitor for include itch, rash, signs of physical dependence.

(Jordan 2008)

5   **Explain how opioid drugs work.**

A   Opioid agonists reduce pain by binding to opiate receptor sites in the peripheral nervous system and the central nervous system (CNS). These mimic the effects of endorphins (naturally occurring opiates that are part of the body's own pain relief system). Endorphins bind to receptors on the peripheral pain neurone to inhibit the release of substance P. When substance P is inhibited, this retards the transmission of pain impulses onto higher centres (the CNS) (Adams et al. 2005).

Following initial investigations, Sam is admitted to a surgical ward. He is continuing to vomit. His pain is now becoming very severe and more widespread. His abdomen is becoming more distended. He appears to be pale and sweaty. His consultant has decided that he will require surgery that evening.

6   **What could be a possible explanation for the further deterioration in his condition?**

A   Increasing abdominal pain and distension can be a sign of peritonitis and perforation of the bowel, demonstrating a deteriorating clinical condition (Hughes 2005).

Following consultation with the doctors, it is decided that Sam should be taken to theatre.

7   **Discuss the key pre-operative care interventions that this patient would require.**

A   • *Pain management*: Administer further opioid analgesia for severe pain. Unfortunately, however, opiates can further compound the experience of nausea and vomiting in patients with bowel obstruction and therefore administration of an anti-emetic, e.g. cyclizine, should also be considered. Metoclopramide is commonly used in surgical settings for the management of nausea and vomiting; however, it is suggested that this drug may be contraindicated in the case of bowel obstruction due to its mode of action. Metoclopramide is said to act as a prokinetic which stimulates gastric emptying. It will therefore further distend the bowel as the stomach contents will pass into an area of the gut where there is no possible outlet. Cyclizine, however, acts on the chemoreceptor trigger zone and/or vomiting centre to block the neurotransmitters and therefore should not further compound the problem of distension (Hughes 2005).

- *Fluid resuscitation*: As Sam is likely to be dehydrated due to diminished absorption of fluids, it is important that fluid and electrolyte levels are corrected and maintained. Administration of appropriate IV fluids is essential, together with hourly fluid balance measurements and careful monitoring to ensure that electrolyte levels are being corrected.
- *Nil by mouth*: As the fluid levels in the gut can rise quickly, this will cause the bowel to become further dilated, preventing absorption of fluids and electrolytes. The patient is therefore at risk of vomiting and thus of aspirating, particularly if going for surgery (Whiteing and Hunter 2008).
- *Nasogastric tube*: Insertion of a nasogastric tube will help to decompress the stomach and therefore reduce the risk and discomfort of vomiting. This will be further aided by regular aspiration of the tube together with the administration of an appropriate anti-emetic (Hughes 2005).

Initial investigations (e.g. X-ray) indicate that Sam has a small bowel obstruction. His vital signs are now:

Temperature: 38.5°C
Pulse: 125 beats per minute
RR: 26 breaths per minute
BP: 85/50 mmHg
U&E results:

	Normal values
Na$^+$: 130 mmol/L	(135–145 mmol/L)
K$^+$: 3.2 mmol/L	(3.5–5.0 mmol/L)
Ca$^+$: 2.2 mmol/L	(2.1–2.6 mmol/L)
Mg: 0.8 mmol/L	(0.75–1.15 mmol/L)
Urea: 1.2 mmol/L	(3.3–8.0 mmol/L)
Creatinine: 120 mmol/L	(40–110 mmol/L)

His white cell count (WCC) is raised at 16x10^9/L (normal range 4–10x10^9/L). The arterial blood gas also indicates a metabolic acidosis.

---

8 **Discuss these observations/blood results and explain why these may be abnormal in relation to the underlying pathophysiology.**

A • *Temperature 38.5°C*: The increased pressure in the intestine tends to compromise mucosal blood flow, which may lead to necrosis and movement of fluids into the luminal fields. This promotes rapid growth of bacteria in the obstructed bowel. Anaerobes grow rapidly in this favourable environment. If perforation does occur, this can rapidly lead to sepsis (Mattson Porth 2007).

- *Pulse increased*: Tachycardia can be linked to the compensatory mechanism associated with hypovolaemia as the heart attempts to circulate the lower blood volume.
- *Respiratory rate increased*: This is increased as the heart and lungs work together to oxygenate the small volume of circulating blood and remove excess carbon dioxide from the blood. It is also worth noting, if distension is severe enough, it may push against the diaphragm and decrease lung volume.
- *Blood pressure low*: The patient may become increasingly hypotensive due to the low circulatory volume.
- *Sodium (Na+) and Potassium (K+) low*: Vomiting can result in severe electrolyte disturbances.
- *Urea and creatinine raised*: Reduced cardiac output to the kidney, due to hypovolaemia, will affect renal perfusion and may lead to acute renal failure.
- *WCC raised*: A raised WCC can be an indicator of infection. This could suggest perforation or even ensuing sepsis and possible bacterial translocation as the gut becomes so distended that the bowel contents are able to pass through its membranes.
- *Metabolic acidosis*: With prolonged obstruction, metabolic acidosis is likely to occur because bicarbonate from pancreatic secretions and bile cannot be absorbed. Hypokalaemia can also occur and could further promote acidosis. Starvation due to the nausea and vomiting can also lead to ketosis, which will further compound the problem of metabolic acidosis. Eventually if pressure from the distension is severe enough, it could lead to strangulation of the arterial circulation and can cause ischaemia, necrosis, perforation, and peritonitis. Lack of circulation permits the build-up of significant amounts of lactic acid, which again will cause the metabolic acidosis to worsen.

Sam is safely transferred to theatre. A bed has been arranged for him in the High Dependency Unit (HDU)/ICU following his surgery where he will hopefully make significant progress to enable him to be transferred back to the ward for on-going care.

Key points

- Alteration in respiratory rate is accepted as being one of the earliest indicators of patient deterioration in the acutely unwell patient.
- Initial management of intestinal obstruction is by fluid and electrolyte resuscitation and the use of a nasogastric tube for aspiration and decompression of the bowel.
- An increase in temperature, pulse rate, pain levels or white cell count will require further investigation as this may indicate a further deterioration in the patient's condition.

REFERENCES

Adams, M.P., Josephson, D.L. and Holland, L.N. (2005) *Pharmacology for Nurses: A Pathophysiologic Approach*. New Jersey: Pearson Education Inc.

Ahern, J. and Philpot, P. (2002) Assessing acutely ill patients on general wards, *Nursing Standard*, 16(47): 47–54.

Baines, M.J. (1997) ABC of palliative care: nausea, vomiting and intestinal obstruction, *British Medical Journal*, 315: 1148–50.

Cole, E., Lynch, A. and Cugnoni, H. (2006) Assessment of the patient with acute abdominal pain, *Nursing Standard*, 20(39): 67–75.

Hughes, E. (2005) Caring for the patient with an intestinal obstruction, *Nursing Standard*, 19(47): 56–64.

Jordan, S. (2008) *The Prescription Guide for Nurses*. Maidenhead: Open University Press.

Longmore, M., Wilkinson, I. and Rajagopalan, S. (2004) *Oxford Handbook of Clinical Medicine*, 6th edn. Oxford: Oxford University Press.

Manterola, C., Vial, M., Moraga, J. and Astudillo, P. (2011) Analgesia in patients with acute abdominal pain (Review). *Cochrane Database of Systematic Reviews*, 3, Art. No. CD005660. Chichester: The Cochrane Collaboration and John Wiley and Sons.

Mattson Porth, C. (2007) *Essentials of Pathophysiology: Concepts of Altered Health States*, 2nd edn. Philadelphia, PA: Lippincott Williams and Wilkins.

NMC (Nursing and Midwifery Council) (2010) *Standards for Medicines Management*. London: NMC.

Smeltzer, S.C., Bare, B.G., Hinkle, J.L. and Cheever, K.H. (2008) *Brunner and Suddarth's Textbook of Medical-Surgical Nursing*, 11th edn. Philadelphia, PA: Lippincott Williams Wilkins.

Whiteing, N. and Hunter, J. (2008) Nursing management of patients who are nil by mouth, *Nursing Standard*, 22(26): 40–5.

Acute pancreatitis
Karen Page

Case outline

Mrs Helen Jones, a 57-year-old woman, was admitted to the acute admissions ward via the A&E unit, complaining of severe epigastric abdominal pain which radiated into her back. She had been out for a meal with her husband and friends the night before; however, soon after they arrived home, she had begun to experience abdominal pain. This had become increasingly severe and she had become nauseated and vomited once prior to admission. Helen was alert and orientated although she was very restless and appeared quite distressed.

An initial ABCDE assessment established the following information:

Temperature: 38.1°C
Pulse: 102 beats per minute
Respiratory rate: 24 breaths per minute
Blood pressure: 118/70 mmHg
Oxygen saturations: 96% on room air
Abdominal tenderness and guarding were noted in the right upper quadrant with diminished bowel sounds present.

---

1   **What additional information with respect to her pain should you establish for Helen at this time?**

A   A systematic approach to assessment and history taking is extremely important to ensure that the patient receives the appropriate treatment for abdominal pain. The PQRST mnemonic is considered to be a useful approach to establish specific information in relation to pain (Cole et al. 2006). This will contribute to establishing the correct diagnosis and planning appropriate interventions.

Check points: PQRST

- *P = Position and radiation.* Abdominal pain can be considered to have three broad categories which can indicate a variety of underlying causes: (1) visceral; (2) parietal; and (3) referred.

- *Visceral pain* is deep, dull and poorly localized and may originate from a solid or hollow structure. It occurs when hollow abdominal organs such as the intestine contract unusually forcefully or are distended or stretched. Solid organs such as the liver can also become painful when their capsule or outer covering is stretched. Visceral pain may be difficult to localize and patients often complain of epigastric pain associated with the stomach, duodenum or pancreas. In practice, the only universal symptom of acute pancreatitis is a continuous, boring, epigastric pain (Kingsnorth and O'Reilly 2006). However, problems in the biliary tree or liver may also cause epigastric pain or pain in the right upper quadrant.
- *Parietal pain* originates in the parietal peritoneum and is caused by inflammation. It is a steady aching pain that is usually more severe than visceral pain and more precisely localized over the involved structure. It is typically aggravated by moving or coughing and patients with this type of pain usually prefer to lie still (Bickley 2007).
- *Referred pain* is felt in more distant sites from the source of the pain, thus pain of pancreatic origin may be referred to the back (Brenner and Krenzer 2010). This occurs because of the anatomical relationships between the affected organ or viscera and associated nerve tracts (Bickley 2007).
- *Q = Quality of the pain.* The patient should be asked to describe the pain using their own words; however, commonly they may use words such as dull, aching, burning, crampy or sharp.
- *R = Relieving or exacerbating factors.* Patients should be asked if something aggravates or relieves the pain e.g. meals, antacids, alcohol, medications such as aspirin, vomiting, passing wind or stools. Eating fatty foods and ingestion of alcohol can often exacerbate the abdominal pain associated with acute pancreatitis (Despins et al. 2005).
- *S = Severity.* A verbal rating score such as the numerical rating scale which asks the patient to rate the pain on a scale from 1–10 is commonly used as it is easy to complete and will allow evaluation of both the initial pain and the effectiveness of any analgesia which is administered.
- *T = Timing and duration.* Careful timing of the pain can be particularly useful. In patients with acute pancreatitis, the pain is usually severe and increases in intensity over a few hours before reaching a plateau that may last for several days (Kingsnorth and O'Reilly 2006).

Helen was experiencing pain which appeared to be originating from the right upper abdominal area on admission which includes a number of important abdominal organs including the pancreas.

---

2   **Briefly consider the normal function of the pancreas to explain why serum amylase and lipase are useful investigations for this patient presenting with acute abdominal pain.**

A   The pancreas is a retroperitoneal organ, situated behind the stomach, stretching from the duodenum to the spleen. It has both endocrine and exocrine functions. The endocrine function of the pancreas is carried out by pancreatic islets (islets of Langerhans) which regulate glucose levels in the blood. The exocrine function of the pancreas is carried out by grape-like clusters of cells called pancreatic acini, which secrete a mixture of fluid and digestive enzymes called pancreatic juice.

The pancreas produces about 1200–1500 mL of pancreatic juice daily. This consists mostly of water, some salts, sodium bicarbonate and several enzymes. The enzymes include a carbohydrate-digesting enzyme known as pancreatic amylase, several protein-digesting enzymes including trypsinogen and chymotrypsinogen, and the principal triglyceride or fat-digesting enzyme in adults, pancreatic lipase. The protein-digesting enzyme trypsin is secreted in an inactive form, trypsinogen, so that it does not digest the cells of the pancreas itself. Pancreatic cells also secrete a trypsin inhibitor that blocks any enzymatic activity in the pancreas. Trypsinogen is normally only converted to trypsin when it comes into contact with the enzyme enterokinase in the small intestine, which then activates the remaining enzymes to facilitate the process of digestion (McCance and Huether 2006).

Although the precise development of pancreatitis is incompletely understood, the most commonly held view is that pancreatitis develops because of injury or disruption to pancreatic acinar cells which permits leakage and premature activation of enzymes into the surrounding pancreatic tissue. In the case of gallstone-related pancreatitis, it is believed that gallstones occlude pancreatic drainage at the level of the ampulla, leading to pancreatic ductal hypertension. This may cause reflux of bile and duodenal contents into the pancreas, leading to premature activation of enzymes and consequent auto-digestion of the pancreatic tissue (Parker 2004). Elevations of the plasma concentrations of pancreatic enzymes are therefore the cornerstones of diagnosis in acute pancreatitis (BSG 2005).

Serum amylase levels rise within 2–12 hours of the onset of symptoms and then gradually return to normal in 3–5 days. If this is measured within 24 hours of the onset of pain, an elevation of three times the upper limit of normal is considered to be indicative of acute pancreatitis. However, raised serum amylase levels are not specific to the pancreas and may be caused by other conditions such as intestinal obstruction, perforation or renal insufficiency. Elevation of isoamylase P is considered to be more specifically related to pancreatic involvement (Brenner and Krenzer 2010). Amylase is rapidly cleared by the kidneys; however, levels of urinary amylase remain elevated for a longer period of time and therefore offer an additional diagnostic investigation (Hughes 2004).

Lipase rises in 4–8 hours, peaks at 24 hours and returns to normal in 8–14 days. Lipase levels at least three times the normal range are considered to be indicative of acute pancreatitis. Simultaneous determination of amylase and lipase levels offers a sensitivity and specificity of between 90% and 95% in establishing a diagnosis of pancreatitis in patients presenting with acute abdominal pain (Parker 2004).

Raised serum amylase and lipase levels indicate that Helen is suffering from acute pancreatitis. Other laboratory tests requested by medical staff included full blood count, liver function tests, urea and electrolytes, coagulation screen, triglycerides, blood glucose, arterial blood gases and C-reactive protein (CRP). A chest X-ray was requested to exclude pleural effusion and an ultrasound scan was performed later that day which demonstrated the presence of gallstones.

3   **Outline the two most common causes of acute pancreatitis.**

A   Gallstones continue to be the most common cause of acute pancreatitis and represent approximately half of the cases with a further 20–25% of cases related to alcohol abuse (BSG 2005). There is concern that the incidence of pancreatitis in the UK appears to be rising due to growing alcohol consumption and an increase in the incidence of gallstones (Kingsnorth and O'Reilly 2006). Helen indicated that she took a glass of wine very occasionally but did not have any alcohol with her meal last night suggesting that gallstones are more likely to be the underlying predisposing cause in this case. The prevalence of gallstones is strongly influenced by age and sex. There is a progressive incidence of gallstones with age but the prevalence is two to three times higher in women than men. The majority of gallstones do not cause any symptoms; however, there is potential for gallstones to cause obstruction and subsequent illness. Numerous other causes of acute pancreatitis including drug-related episodes have been described which account for the remaining cases of the disease.

4   **Following a diagnosis of acute pancreatitis due to gallstones, what interventions need to be considered for this patient? Consider the nurse's role in relation to these.**

A   Conventional care of the patient with acute pancreatitis focuses on pain management, ensuring adequate levels of oxygenation, fluid and electrolyte replacement, providing nutritional support and early detection and treatment of complications such as pancreatic necrosis, sepsis or organ dysfunction. The role of the nurse is to deliver essential nursing care, monitor the patient closely and promptly identify and highlight any improvement or deterioration in the patient's condition.

NURSING INTERVENTIONS

Pain management

Acute pancreatic pain increases metabolic activity which in turn increases the release of pancreatic enzymes and therefore effective pain management is critical to sustain comfort, decrease anxiety and promote recovery (Burruss and Holz 2005).

- Assess the patient's pain regularly using a valid and reliable pain assessment tool.
- Administer the prescribed analgesia as required. An opioid drug such as morphine is usually required to manage the severe pain associated with acute pancreatitis.
- Monitor for effects/side effects associated with opioid drugs.
- Provide additional measures of pain relief such as reassurance, information and positioning to help to minimize the pain.

Alleviate nausea and vomiting

Pain is often accompanied by nausea and vomiting in acute pancreatitis; however, no relief of abdominal pain is achieved by vomiting. In addition, prolonged or excess vomiting may lead to dehydration which can exacerbate the symptoms of hypovolaemia which are associated with the development of the acute inflammatory process in pancreatitis.

- Minimize pancreatic stimulation by maintaining nil by mouth status.
- Administer prescribed anti-emetic drugs regularly and monitor for effectiveness.
- If the patient has reduced or absent bowel sounds, indicating paralytic ileus, the use of a nasogastric tube may help to decompress the stomach and provide some pain relief (Holcomb 2007).
- Consider nasogastric feeding if resumption of oral intake is delayed to maintain nutritional status.

Oxygen therapy

Providing adequate oxygen therapy is essential when treating patients with acute pancreatitis who are at risk of organ failure. Oxygen saturations below 95% or changes in the patient's baseline respiratory rate indicate increased oxygen requirements or decreased respiratory function. A chest X-ray will demonstrate the presence of any pleural effusion caused by auto-digestion of lung tissue from the passage of pancreatic exudates via the lymph channels to the chest or movement of inflammatory exudates through the diaphragm.

- Monitor and record level of consciousness, respiratory rate, pulse oximetry. Any signs of deterioration should be reported immediately to the appropriate healthcare personnel.
- Monitor arterial blood gases. Impaired insulin secretion as a result of pancreatic necrosis, releases large quantities of fatty acids into the circulation. These are converted into ketones, causing metabolic acidosis. Pancreatitis also reduces levels of bicarbonate which may cause blood pH to drop further (Parker 2004).
- Supplemental oxygen should be administered as prescribed to maintain oxygen saturation greater than 95% (Brenner and Krenzer 2010).
- Chest physiotherapy and appropriate positioning will assist in optimizing ventilation.

Fluid resuscitation

The release of inflammatory mediators following autodigestion of the pancreatic tissue causes alterations in capillary permeability. This permits large fluid losses into the extravascular space and peritoneal cavity, leading to the risk of hypovolaemic shock and hypotension. The first goal of treatment therefore is to stabilize the patient haemodynamically. As it is difficult on admission to predict which patients will develop complications, it is appropriate to ensure that all patients with acute pancreatitis receive suitable fluid resuscitation early in the disease process until it is clear that the danger of hypovolaemia leading to organ failure has passed (BSG 2005).

- Establish IV access as soon as possible using wide-bore peripheral cannula.
- Administer intravenous fluids (crystalloid or colloid) as prescribed based on the results of laboratory tests e.g. haematocrit, haemoglobin, urea and electrolytes, serum albumin.

- Monitor and record the patient's response to IV fluid therapy including pulse, blood pressure and capillary refill. The use of an early warning score (EWS) will allow early recognition and reporting of changes in clinical parameters (NICE 2007). Central venous pressure recording may be required if substantial fluid resuscitation is indicated.
- Monitor and record urinary output to ensure that this is >0.5 mL/kg/hour, indicating adequate renal perfusion.

Electrolyte disturbances

Persistent vomiting may result in hypokalaemia. Hypocalcaemia may indicate the presence of pancreatic fat necrosis because calcium binds with fatty acids during tissue necrosis. In addition, trypsin inactivates parathyroid hormone (PTH) which is needed for calcium absorption (McCance and Huether 2006).

- Monitor ECG to ensure that patients remain in sinus rhythm.
- Monitor serum urea and electrolyte levels. Advise medical staff if results are outside normal range.

Hyperglycaemia can occur as the result of impaired insulin secretion from damaged pancreatic beta cells, increased glucagon release, and increased levels of catecholamines.

- Monitor blood glucose levels regularly
- Administer insulin as prescribed to maintain blood sugar levels within the normal range.

5 **Consider the nursing care required by Helen while she is receiving nil by mouth.**

A Oral hygiene is an essential nursing intervention that should be considered a priority for any patient who is receiving nil by mouth yet it is suggested many patients do not receive adequate mouth care while in hospital (Evans 2001). When patients are unable to eat or drink, the mouth becomes dry and the nurse needs to provide adequate oral hygiene to keep the mouth clean and reduce the risk of potential infection. In addition, patients may require oxygen therapy that will also dry the mouth and cause discomfort. Patients should therefore be offered regular mouthwashes and given the appropriate equipment to allow them to carry out their own oral care if they are fit to do so. In the event that the patient cannot be self-caring in this respect, the nurse must ensure regular mouth care to maintain the health of the oral cavity. A lip lubricant may also be appropriate to moisten the lips, prevent cracking and help provide a natural barrier for potential infection (Xavier 2000).

It must also be remembered that along with the physical problems associated with nil by mouth status, the patient may also suffer psychological distress. The nurse must ensure that she explains carefully in a clear and concise way the rationale for any proposed nil by mouth decision and this should help to go some way towards addressing the patient's needs (Whiteing and Hunter 2008).

6 **What criteria can be used to predict the severity of an episode of pancreatitis?**

A Acute pancreatitis is self-limiting and mild in the majority of patients and will resolve spontaneously within 5–7 days (Morton and Fontaine 2009). However, in 10–20% of patients, acute pancreatitis is a severe and potentially fatal disease and results in systemic inflammatory responses (sepsis) and progressive multi-organ failure. Early identification of the severity of an attack is important as it facilitates appropriate transfer to critical care if required to decrease complications and reduce mortality.

Severity of pancreatitis is measured using different scoring methods (Table 11.1). The Ranson score comprises five clinical criteria measured on admission and six clinical criteria measured at 48 hours. The criteria measured on admission reflect the local inflammatory effects of pancreatic enzymes; those measured at 48 hours represent the later systemic effects. Three or more Ranson criteria demonstrated within 48 hours predict severe pancreatitis and should prompt intensive care for the patient (Despins et al. 2005). The modified Glasgow criterion is the easiest and quickest way to evaluate the severity of pancreatitis (Imrie 1975). Severe disease is considered to be present if three or more factors are detected within 48 hours. The APACHE (acute physiology, age, chronic health evaluation) score is generated from multiple parameters and is considered highly accurate. In addition, it allows

Table 11.1 Scoring systems to measure acute pancreatitis

Ranson's criteria for severity of acute pancreatitis	Modified Glasgow criteria (assessed at 48 hours)	The APACHE 11 scoring system parameters
On Admission	*On Admission*	*Physiological*
Age >55 years	Age >55 years	Mean arterial pressure
WCC >16,000/mm^3	WCC 15,000/mm^3	Temperature
Blood glucose >10 mmol/L	Blood glucose >10 mmol/L	Heart rate
AST >250 IU/L	BUN level >16mmol/L	Respiratory rate
LDH >350 IU/L	LDH >600 IU/L	Glasgow Coma Scale
After 48 hours	Calcium <2 mmol/L	*Laboratory*
Haematocrit drop >10%	Albumin <32 g/L	Arterial pH/P_aO_2
BUN increase >10 mmol/L	PaO_2<8.0kPa	Serum sodium
PaO_2<8.0 kPa	Score 1 point for each criteria met	Serum potassium
Base deficit >4 mEq/L		Serum creatinine
Calcium <2 mmol/L	(Imrie 1975)	Haematocrit
Estimated fluid needs >6 L		White cell count
1 point for each criteria met		Score 0–4 (normal to abnormal)
(Ranson 1985)		Adjust for age, severe organ insufficiency, immunocompromise
		BMI is an additional parameter
		(Kumar and Clarke 2005)

AST aspartate aninotransferase; BUN blood urea nitrogen; LDH Lactate dehydrogenase.

prediction of severity as early as 24 hours from the onset of symptoms; however, this scoring system is more time-consuming. Clinical assessment of increased severity includes signs of haemodynamic instability or organ failure, BMI over 30, and an APACHE 11 score greater than 8 (Kumar and Clarke 2005).

C-reactive protein (CRP), an acute phase protein produced by the liver, has been shown to reflect the degree of inflammatory insult and therefore CRP levels can assist in predicting a severe attack. Unfortunately CRP does not become significantly elevated until 48 hours after inflammation, limiting its use in the diagnosis of acute pancreatitis. However, CRP levels greater than 130 mg/L within the first 72 hours of acute pancreatitis have correlated with the presence of pancreatic necrosis with sensitivity of greater than 80% (BSG 2005).

In addition to these scoring systems, computed tomography (CT) scanning can demonstrate inflammation, fluid collection and changes consistent with pancreatic necrosis. In general, the more complex the symptoms revealed by the CT scan, the more likely the patient will be to suffer a more severe attack (Balthazar 2002; Koo et al. 2010).

Helen had a Glasgow score of 2, 48 hours following admission. Her condition resolved with supportive treatment and she began oral intake again on day 4 of her in-patient stay. She was discharged on a low fat diet with an appointment to return to the outpatient clinic the following week. As the patient was diagnosed with gallstones, she was advised that she would require a cholecystectomy as soon as possible to prevent reccurrence of acute pancreatitis.

Key points

- Pancreatitis should be considered in patients presenting with acute epigastric pain.
- Serum amylase and lipase are useful diagnostic investigations in acute pancreatitis.
- Pancreatitis can have serious complications. Constant monitoring for evidence of any deterioration in the patient's condition is essential.

REFERENCES

Balthazar, E.J. (2002) Assessment of severity with clinical and CT evaluation, *Radiology*, 223: 603–12.

Bickley, L.S. (2007) *Bates Guide to Physical Examination and History Taking*, 9th edn. Philadelphia, PA: Lippincott Williams and Wilkins.

Brenner, Z.R. and Krenzer, M.E. (2010) Understanding acute pancreatitis, *Nursing*, January, pp. 32–9.

BSG (British Society of Gastroenterology) (2005) UK guidelines for the management of acute pancreatitis: UK Working Party on Acute Pancreatitis, *Gut*, 54(Suppl. 3): iii, 1–9.

Burruss, N. and Holz, S. (2005) Understanding acute pancreatitis, *Nursing*, 35(3): 32–4.

Cole, E., Lynch, A. and Cugnoni, H. (2006) Assessment of the patient with acute abdominal pain, *Nursing Standard*, 20(39): 67–75.

Despins, L., Kivlahan, C. and Cox, K. (2005) Acute pancreatitis: diagnosis and treatment of a potentially fatal condition, *American Journal of Nursing*, 105(11): 54–47.

Evans, G. (2001) A rationale for oral care, *Nursing Standard*, 15(43): 33–6.

Holcomb, S.S. (2007) Stopping the destruction of acute pancreatitis, *Nursing*, June: 43–8.

Hughes, E. (2004) Understanding the care of patients with acute pancreatitis. *Nursing Standard*, 18(18): 45–52.

Imrie, C.W. (1975) A prospective study of acute pancreatitis, *British Journal of Surgery*, 62(6): 490–4.

Kingsnorth, A. and O'Reilly, D. (2006) Acute pancreatitis, *British Medical Journal*, 332: 1072–6.

Koo, B.C., Chinogureyi, A. and Shaw, A.S. (2010) Imaging acute pancreatitis, *The British Journal of Radiology*, 83: 104–12.

Kumar, P. and Clark, M. (2005) *Clinical Medicine*, 6th edn. London: Elsevier Saunders.

McCance, K.L. and Huether, S.E. (2006) *Pathophysiology: The Biologic Basis for Disease in Adults and Children*, 5th edn. St Louis, MO: Elsevier Mosby.

Morton, P.G. and Fontaine, D.K. (2009) *Critical Care Nursing: A Holistic Approach*, 9th edn. Philadelphia, PA: Lippincott Williams and Wilkins.

NICE (National Institute for Health and Clinical Excellence) (2007) *Acutely Ill Patients in Hospital: Recognition of and Response to Acute Illness in Adults in Hospital*. Clinical Guideline No. 50. London: NICE.

Parker, M. (2004) Acute pancreatitis, *Emergency Nurse*, 11(10): 28–35.

Ranson, J.H.C. (1985) Risk factors in acute pancreatitis, *Hospital Practice (Office Ed.)*, 20(4): 69–73.

Whiteing, N. and Hunter, J. (2008) Nursing management of patients who are nil by mouth, *Nursing Standard*, 22(26): 40–5.

Xavier, G. (2000) The importance of mouth care in preventing infection, *Nursing Standard*, 14(18): 47–51.

PART 6
Endocrine System

Diabetic ketoacidosis
Karen Page

Case outline

Susan, a 22-year-old woman who was known to have type 1 diabetes, was admitted to the acute medical ward by her GP, following a home visit as she was feeling very unwell. An initial ABCDE assessment of the patient revealed the following information: Susan was orientated and able to respond to questions indicating a patent airway although she was quite lethargic.

Respiratory rate: 26 breaths/minute (rapid and shallow)
Blood pressure: 100/65 mmHg
Pulse: 105 beats per minute (regular)
Temperature 36.5°C
Oxygen saturations: 96% on room air

Susan gave a history of four episodes of vomiting accompanied by abdominal pain over the past 24 hours. She was not tolerating food or fluid at present although she complained of thirst. On examination, dry mucous membranes were apparent. An abdominal examination revealed diffuse abdominal pain – pain score 6/10 constant, non-radiating, with no aggravating or relieving factors.

Chest X-ray revealed no obvious abnormalities.
Urinalysis was positive for ketones +++, glucose ++++ with evidence of possible infection.
Capillary blood glucose level 30.7 mmol/L.
ABG reveals evidence of acidosis

---

1   **Provide an outline of normal blood glucose homeostasis.**

A   Insulin and glucagon are the key hormones involved in the storage and controlled release within the body of the chemical energy available from food. These hormones are synthesized in the alpha cells (glucagon) and beta cells (insulin) of the pancreatic islets of Langerhans and are critical in the regulation of blood sugar levels within the range of 4.0–8.0 mmol/L. Following a meal, insulin is secreted in response to higher blood sugar levels. This facilitates an increased rate of uptake of glucose by many cells within the body, including the liver, muscle and adipose tissue and stimulates the production of fats and proteins. The net effect of this is to decrease blood glucose levels. When blood sugar levels fall, glucagon stimulates the liver to release glucose, either by converting stored glycogen to glucose, or by the process of gluconeogenesis which produces glucose from amino acids and glycerol to maintain blood sugar levels (Hassell and Butler-Williams 2010).

2   **Discuss the precipitating factors associated with diabetic ketoacidosis (DKA).**

A   Ketoacidosis may be the initial presentation of type 1 diabetes or it may be associated with other precipitating factors such as the stress of intercurrent infection or trauma. Management errors such as inappropriate changes in dosage regime or dosage errors, discontinuation or erratic compliance with insulin have also been noted (Jerreat 2010). This is often because the patient feels unable to eat due to nausea or vomiting and assumes that if they are eating less, they should decrease their insulin dosage. However, the deliberate omission of insulin as a result of a fear of weight gain is also a common cause of diabetic ketoacidosis, particularly in young women who may also suffer from clinically significant eating disorders (Kumar and Clark 2005; Kitabchi et al. 2006). Recreational drugs and alcoholic binges have also been shown to precipitate ketoacidosis in individuals with type 1 diabetes (Lee et al. 2009; Jerreat 2010).

3   **Susan is demonstrating features associated with DKA including hyperglycaemia, ketonaemia and acidosis. Provide an explanation of the pathological changes which have contributed to these clinical features.**

A   Table 12.1 presents the pathological changes associated with DKA.

Table 12.1 Pathological changes associated with DKA

Change	Description
Hyperglycaemia Raised blood sugar >11 mmol/L	Diabetes type 1 results from insulin deficiency; however, considerable evidence suggests that both alpha cell and beta cell production are abnormal and that both a lack of insulin and a relative excess of glucagon exist. As the insulin-sensitive tissues are deprived of glucose, the body reacts by increasing production of counter-regulatory hormones, i.e. glucagon, catecholamines (epinephrine and norepine-phrine), cortisol and growth hormone. This hormonal imbalance increases insulin resistance, leading to decreased cellular uptake of glucose in peripheral tissues. Moreover, it promotes excessive hepatic glucose production (gluconeogenesis) and glycogenolysis. This results in the severe *hyperglycaemia* that occurs in uncontrolled diabetes (Kumar and Clark 2005)
Glycosuria	Glucose is filtered by the renal glomeruli where in the presence of normal blood volume and plasma glucose levels all the glucose is reabsorbed into the bloodstream. When the blood sugar exceeds the normal renal threshold, glucose begins to escape into the urine as the reabsorption capacity of the renal tubules is exceeded (*glycosuria*)

Polyuria	*Polyuria* occurs as a result of the subsequent osmotic diuresis resulting in dehydration, thirst, headache and lethargy. Patients may not be able to drink sufficient water to compensate for the diuresis, which in turn reduces urinary glucose losses and permits the blood glucose level to rise even further. This loss of fluid volume may be demonstrated in a significant drop in blood pressure (*hypotension*). The loss of water is accompanied by a loss of electrolytes including sodium, potassium and chloride. As the excretion of potassium by the kidney occurs through the exchange of potassium for sodium, adequate sodium may not be available to facilitate this mechanism leading to the potential for high levels of serum potassium (Smeltzer et al. 2008)
Ketonaemia	Lipolysis occurs because of the deficit in available insulin and the enhanced effects of counter-regulatory hormones which allow activation of lipase, the key regulator of the breakdown of fat stores (Jerreat 2010). Lipolysis increases the production of free fatty acids which are then metabolized within the liver to provide an alternative energy source, resulting in accumulation of the end metabolite –
Moderate ketonuria or blood ketone levels above 3 mmol/L	ketone bodies. Ketones include acetone, acetoactetate and the predominant ketone found in DKA 3-beta-hydroxybutyrate (Wallace and Matthews 2004). These excess ketones are excreted via the kidney resulting in *ketonuria*
	The presence of ketones induces anorexia, nausea, vomiting and abdominal pain which further exacerbates fluid and electrolyte loss. A variety of compensatory mechanisms are therefore initiated to prevent vascular collapse and shock. One such mechanism is an increase in
Fluid depletion	pulse rate (*tachycardia*) which attempts to maintain cardiac output in the face of shrinking vascular volume. On average, body water is depleted by 5–6 litres in DKA (Morton and Fontaine 2009)
	If these ketones are produced faster than they can be used or excreted, it will lead to the development of a metabolic acidosis. In an attempt to correct this acidosis *hyperventilation* occurs to expel excess carbon dioxide gas. This increase in breathing is gradual at first; however, *Kussmaul's respirations* are associated with a gradual increase in the depth rather than the frequency of respirations and are characteristic of a severe degree of acidosis
Acidosis Significant acidosis, e.g. bicarbonate ≤15 mmol/L or pH <7.3	in DKA. Excess ketones also appear in breath and are associated with the classic fruity 'peardrop' odour found in DKA (Kumar and Clark 2005)
	The diminished vascular volume leads to a decrease in tissue perfusion. The resulting decrease in oxygen causes these tissues to shift from aerobic to anaerobic respiration, leading to increased production of lactic acid. This further aggravates the already existing metabolic acidosis

4 **Explain how Susan's blood gas results confirm the presence of a metabolic acidosis.**

A Susan's blood gas results were:

Blood gas results	Normal range
Bicarbonate (HCO_3^-) 10.0 mmol/L	24–28 mmol/L
pH 7.26	7.35–7.45
$PaCO_2$ 3.15 kPa	4.65–6.0 kPa
PaO_2 12.55 kPa	10.5–14.0 kPa

Metabolic acidosis is a clinical disturbance characterized by low pH, and loss of bicarbonate (HCO_3). Plasma pH is in fact an indicator of hydrogen (H^+) ion concentration. H^+ ion concentration is extremely important since the greater the concentration, the more acidic the solution and the lower the pH. Conversely, the lower the H^+ ion concentration, the more alkaline the solution and the higher the pH will be. Homeostatic mechanisms keep the pH within a normal range. These mechanisms consist of buffer systems, the kidneys and the lungs. Buffer systems prevent major changes in the pH of body fluids by either removing or releasing hydrogen. The body's major extracellular buffer system is the bicarbonate-carbonic acid system which is assessed when blood gases are measured. Normally there are 20 parts of bicarbonate (an alkali) to one part of carbonic acid; however, if this ratio is altered, the pH will change. As ketoacids enter the extracellular fluid, the H^+ ion is removed and neutralized by combining with bicarbonate in an effort to maintain the pH within normal limits (Morton and Fontaine 2009). Low levels of bicarbonate are therefore caused by extensive buffering to maintain plasma pH levels. The lungs control carbon dioxide (CO_2) levels and therefore the carbonic acid content of the plasma. They do so by adjusting ventilation in response to the amount of CO_2 in the blood. In metabolic acidosis, the respiratory rate increases, causing greater elimination of CO_2 to reduce the acid load (Smeltzer et al. 2008).

Obtaining an arterial blood gas sample from an artery is painful and carries the risk of damage to the artery. Recent evidence shows that the difference between venous and arterial pH is 0.02–0.15 pH units and the difference between arterial and venous bicarbonate is 1.88 mmol/L (Gokel et al. 2000; Kelly 2006). As this will change neither the diagnosis nor management of DKA, it is not always considered necessary to use arterial blood to measure acid–base status (Ma et al. 2003; Jerreat 2010). The pH and HCO_3^- are both significantly reduced in Susan's blood gas, indicating the presence of a metabolic acidosis. The $PaCO_2$ is reduced, resulting from a respiratory effort to try to compensate for the metabolic acidosis.

5 **Consider the treatment regime Susan will require to manage her current episode of DKA.**

A Ketoacidosis is an acute complication which occurs primarily but not exclusively in patients with type 1 diabetes and results in the patient becoming acutely ill. It must be treated as a medical emergency due to the potential morbidity and mortality which are associated with this condition. Many of these patients are managed in acute medical areas, therefore the nurse must ensure that she is familiar with the management of DKA (Figure 12.1). It involves fluid replacement, insulin replacement and correction of electrolyte disturbances.

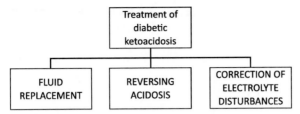

Figure 12.1 Treatment of diabetic ketoacidosis

NURSING INTERVENTIONS

Fluid replacement

Rehydration of patients with intravenous fluid replacement is essential in patients with DKA. The aim is to restore circulatory volume and maintain tissue perfusion. Fluid resuscitation will also assist in the clearance of excess glucose and ketones and correct electrolyte disturbances.

Crystalloid rather than colloid solutions are recommended for fluid replacement. The hypotension that occurs in DKA results from a loss of an electrolyte solution and a recent Cochrane Review (Perel and Roberts 2007) supported the use of a crystalloid solution. It is therefore recommended that 0.9% sodium chloride should be used for fluid resuscitation in clinical practice as it is readily available in all clinical areas.

Susan has no accompanying disease processes; however, caution is required with older adults, in those patients who have cardiac or renal disease, those with mild DKA (plasma bicarbonate >10 mmol/L) or pregnancy. More rapid infusion rates may increase the risk of respiratory distress syndrome (Jerreat 2010).

Correction of electrolyte disturbances

Hypokalaemia and hyperkalaemia are potentially life-threatening conditions associated with DKA. Serum potassium is often high on admission but can fall rapidly on administration of insulin. Insulin facilitates the intracellular transport of potassium and is crucial to the regulation of serum potassium levels. It is therefore essential to monitor serum potassium levels as the level will almost always fall as insulin therapy is commenced (Morton and Fontaine 2009). Moreover rehydration leads to increased plasma volume and subsequent decreases in the concentration of serum potassium with increased urinary excretion of potassium. Potassium can be transfused with 0.9% sodium chloride solution and is available in ready mixed solutions (20 mmol/L KCl, 40 mmol/L KCl) which supports safe practice and complies with medicine safety alerts where potassium addition in general clinical areas is recognized as being associated with significant risk (NPSA 2002, 2009).

Reversing acidosis

Blood glucose may fall very rapidly as insulin is administered to correct ketoacidosis and it is essential not to allow hypoglycaemia to develop. This may result in a rebound ketosis driven by counter-regulatory hormones (JBDS 2010). Once the blood glucose falls to ≤15 mmol/L, intravenous glucose 10% must be commenced to prevent hypoglycaemia (Jerreat 2010).

JBDS (2010) suggest that a stat. dose of soluble insulin intramuscularly (IM) is only given if venous access is proving difficult or a delay in setting up the insulin infusion is anticipated. However, local protocols may advise the administration of an initial bolus dose of insulin prior to a cont-inuous infusion of regular insulin. If the patient is on long-acting insulin, e.g. Lantus, it is recommended that this is continued while the patient is receiving treatment for DKA to provide a basal level of insulin when IV insulin is stopped (JBDS 2010).

Susan was therefore commenced on the following fluid replacement regime:

1 litre 0.9% sodium chloride over 1 hour.
1 litre 0.9% sodium chloride with 20 mmol/KCl over the next two hours.
1 litre 0.9% sodium chloride with 20 mmol/KCl over the next two hours.
1 litre 0.9% sodium chloride with 20 mmol/KCl over the next four hours.

When blood glucose levels are below 14/15 mmol/L, add 1 litre 10% dextrose and reduce the rate of the insulin infusion.

Susan was prescribed 50 units of soluble insulin (Actrapid) made up to 50 mL to be administered as a continuous fixed rate IV infusion via an infusion pump.

Prescribed rate 0.1 unit/kg/hr = 6 mL/hr (Susan's weight – 60 kg).

Note that local policy guidelines and protocols for management of DKA may vary in response to e.g. age or concurrent illness.

---

6 **Highlight the nursing management strategies associated with administration of this therapy.**

- Weigh the patient on admission if their condition allows or alternatively estimate their weight as accurately as possible to facilitate fluid and insulin dosage calculation.
- Label and ensure the insulin is checked and signed for against the prescription as per local policy and the infusion pump is correctly primed.
- Regularly check the insulin infusion pump is connected and working correctly and that the exact insulin residual volume is present to detect any pump malfunction and ensure safe and effective administration of medication.
- Maintain an accurate fluid balance chart to monitor the patient's response to treatment.
- Observe urinary output closely to ensure a minimum of 0.5 mL/kg/hr to observe for adequate renal function.
- Insert nasogastric tube if vomiting persists and administer anti-emetic as prescribed. Provide oral hygiene as required to ensure patient comfort.
- Ensure bedside blood glucose monitoring equipment is maintained correctly and calibrated regularly to facilitate accurate measurements. Staff training should be undertaken on a regular basis to update skills and knowledge on the use of blood glucose measurement tools.

- Record and report capillary blood sugar levels *HOURLY* (recheck laboratory glucose after 2 hours).
- If meter reads blood glucose over 20 mmol/L or Hi, venous blood should be sent to the laboratory or measured using a blood gas analyser until the capillary blood glucose meter is within range to ensure accurate measurements.
- Record and report blood or urinary ketone levels as available *HOURLY*.
- The presence of ketones is the hallmark of DKA. The availability of meters which measure the ketone 3-beta-hydroxybutyrate is a relatively new development; however, there is evidence to support the use of this technology in clinical practice (Sheikh-Ali et al. 2008; JBDS 2010). The resolution of DKA depends on the suppression of ketonaemia and therefore measurement of blood ketones represents best practice in monitoring the response to treatment (JBDS 2010).
- Check *2 HOURLY* serum potassium, pH and bicarbonate level for the first 6 hours and then 4 hourly until stable as potassium levels may drop quickly as a result of rehydration and insulin replacement therapy.
- Monitor ECG for arrhythmias to ensure there are no signs of hyperkalaemia (tall, peaked or tented T waves) (Smeltzer et al. 2008).
- Record regular observations of respiratory rate, BP, pulse, temperature, oxygen saturations, neurological observations, pain score and complete EWS charts to monitor response to treatment and facilitate early detection of any potential complications.
- Establish any precipitating cause – obtain blood cultures, urine cultures and other laboratory specimens as indicated.
- Consider repositioning, deep breathing and leg exercises to reduce the risk of any complications due to reduced mobility.
- Provide assistance with activities of living such as personal hygiene as required to maintain patient comfort.
- Provide reassurance and support to both patient and relatives. Ensure that the purpose of all treatment is explained to the patient and consent to treatment is obtained. An episode of DKA can be a frightening experience and the nurse must work calmly and efficiently to support the patient during assessment and treatment.

Susan responded well to treatment and her physiological parameters began to revert to normal. She began eating and drinking oral fluids when the acidosis had resolved and blood glucose was within normal range. A subcutaneous insulin regime was commenced prior to discontinuing the IV infusion of insulin, and she continued to make satisfactory progress. She was also commenced on antibiotics to treat a urinary tract infection which was detected following admission to the ward.

---

7   **Outline guidelines to assist Susan in the prevention of a recurrence of DKA.**

A   Treatment is considered to be incomplete without identification of the precipitating cause of the episode, e.g. infection or omission of insulin injections. Failure to find this out often represents a missed educational opportunity with the patient so as Susan begins to recover, the nurse must reassess the factors which led to the development of this episode of DKA. On questioning Susan, it was apparent that she had not realized the importance of following the guidelines which should be implemented during periods of illness –'sick day rules'. It is also important for the nurse to check that the patient can accurately use portable blood glucose or ketone measurement devices and correctly self-administer insulin. Susan should also have the opportunity to discuss any concerns or queries with the diabetic nurse specialist prior to discharge who will provide further detailed information and a point of contact when the patient returns home.

ADJUSTING DIABETES MANAGEMENT DURING PERIODS OF ILLNESS

Any illnesses such as common cold, flu, urinary infections, stomach upsets, sore throats or bronchitis, can affect diabetes control. The overriding principle in managing concurrent illness is to prevent escalating blood sugar levels, therefore guidelines for blood glucose management known as 'sick day rules' should be discussed with the patient. These will vary in respect to local protocols; however, they should include the following key principles:

- Normal insulin should never be stopped even if you are not eating or drinking very much. Withholding carbohydrates because of high blood glucose levels may make ketosis worse.
- If you are unable to eat a normal diet, alternative foods/drinks should be substituted. A list of suitable alternatives should be discussed with the patient.
- Test and record blood sugars every 3–4 hours.
- Try to drink plenty of liquids (3–4 litres per day) such as water or sugar-free squash, especially if blood glucose is high.
- If blood sugars rise above 15 mmol/L or you are feeling nauseous, have been sick or have abdominal discomfort, test your urine or blood for ketones. When blood glucose is above 15 mmol/L and urine or blood ketones are present, it is likely that you will require supplemental insulin doses. Contact your GP or diabetes specialist nurse for advice.
- Tell a friend or relative, if you are on your own, that you are ill, and ask them to check on you every 4–6 hours.
- Contact your GP or diabetes specialist nurse for advice as you may require hospital admission when:
  - you have persistent vomiting/stomach pain;
  - you are unable to eat or drink;
  - your illness is not improving;
  - you have high blood glucose levels with or without urinary or blood ketones.

(Smeltzer et al. 2008)

Susan made good progress following treatment of this episode of DKA and was reviewed by the specialist diabetic team prior to discharge. She acknowledged that she wanted to learn more about her condition to prevent further episodes of DKA as she had not realized that this could be so serious. An appointment was made with the diabetic nurse specialist for further follow-up advice after discharge.

Key points
- Regular blood sugar monitoring is key to preventing DKA.
- Features associated with DKA include hyperglycaemia, ketonaemia and acidosis.
- Treatment requires fluid and electrolyte replacement to correct the acidosis present with concurrent insulin therapy.

REFERENCES

Gokel, Y., Paydas, S., Koseoglu, Z., Alparslan, N. and Sydaoglu, G. (2000) Comparison of blood gas and acid-base measurements on arterial and venous blood samples in patients with uremic acidosis and diabetic ketoacidosis in the emergency room, *American Journal of Nephrology*, 4: 319–23.

Hassell, S. and Butler-Williams, C. (2010) Blood sugar monitoring in critically ill patients, *British Journal of Neuroscience Nursing*, 6(7): 342–4.

JBDS (Joint British Diabetes Societies Inpatient Care Group) (2010) *The Management of Diabetic Ketoacidosis in Adults*. London: NHS Diabetes.

Jerreat, L. (2010) Managing diabetic ketoacidosis, *Nursing Standard*, 24(34): 49–55.

Kelly, A.M. (2006) The case for venous rather than arterial blood gases in diabetic ketoacidosis, *Emergency Medicine Australasia*, 18: 64–7.

Kitabchi, A.E., Umpierrez, G.E., Murphy, M.B. and Kriesberg, R.A. (2006) Hyperglycaemic crisis in adult patients with diabetes: a consensus statement from the American Diabetes Association, *Diabetes Care*, 29(12): 2739–48.

Kumar, P. and Clark, M. (2005) *Clinical Medicine*, 6th edn. London: Elsevier Saunders.

Lee, P., Greenfield, J.R. and Campbell, L.V. (2009) Managing young people with Type 1 diabetes in a 'rave' new world: metabolic complications of substance abuse in Type 1 diabetes, *Diabetic Medicine*, 26(4): 328–33.

Ma, O.J., Rush, M.D., Godfrey, M.M. and Gaddis, G. (2003) Arterial blood gas results rarely influence emergency physician management of patients with suspected diabetic ketoacidosis, *Academy of Emergency Medicine*, 8: 836–41.

Morton, P.G. and Fontaine, D.K. (2009) *Critical Care Nursing: A Holistic Approach*, 9th edn. Philadelphia, PA: Lippincott Williams and Wilkins.

NPSA (National Patient Safety Association) (2002) *Patient Safety Alert Potassium Solutions: Risks to Patients from Errors Occurring during Intravenous Administration*. London: NPSA.

NPSA (National Patient Safety Association) (2009) *National Reporting and Learning System (NRLS) Never Events Framework 2009/10*. London: NPSA.

Perel, P. and Roberts, I. (2007) Colloids versus crystalloids for fluid resuscitation in critically ill patients, *Cochrane Database of Systematic Reviews*, Issue 3, Art. No. CD000567.

Sheikh-Ali, M., Karon, B.S., Basu, A. et al. (2008) Can serum beta-hydroxybutyrate be used to diagnose diabetic ketoacidosis? *Diabetes Care*, 4: 643–7.

Smeltzer, S.C., Bare, B., Hinkle, J.L. and Cheever, K.H. (2008) *Brunner and Suddarth's Textbook of Medical-Surgical Nursing*, 11th edn. Philadelphia, PA: Lippincott Williams and Wilkins.

Wallace, T.M. and Matthews, D.R. (2004) Recent advances in the monitoring and management of diabetic ketoacidosis, *Quarterly Journal of Medicine*, 97(12): 773–80.

PART 7
Musculoskeletal System

Acute trauma – fracture
Niall McKenna

Case outline

You are a nurse working in A&E and have received a call from ambulance control to alert the department of the expected arrival of a 23-year-old male (John Brown), who has sustained multiple trauma in a road traffic collision. Estimated time of arrival is 5 minutes.

---

1 **What action must be taken to prepare the department for the arrival of the casualty?**

A Preparation of the admitting environment is essential to allow for the effective evaluation and stabilization of those presenting with trauma injury (Dandy and Edwards 2009).
Action to be taken may include the following;

- Contact relevant medical/surgical personnel – surgical registrar/consultant, anaesthetics, radiology department, laboratory staff/blood bank, administration staff (notes/charts), and portering staff.
- Team briefing to ensure each member knows what task he/she is responsible for.
- Selection of medical staff and nursing team leaders.
- Put on protective clothing.
- Organize airway management equipment, IV fluid preparation.
- Organize oxygen/suction therapy.
- Final check on equipment – pumps, monitors (minimal preparation is necessary).
- Prepare resuscitation trolley.
- Ensure keys to medicine cupboards/fridges are readily available.
- Inform non-urgent cases of extended waiting times.

2 **Outline the assessment/investigations required to establish the patient's status on arrival to the resuscitation room. Provide a rationale for your responses.**

A Rapid assessment utilizing the ABCDE approach is required (Table 13.1).

Table 13.1 The ABCDE procedure for rapid assessment

Assessment/investigations	Rationale
Obtain history and interventions undertaken in the pre-hospital setting	Establishing pertinent history and clinical presentation will assist clinicians in the triage process and guide immediate treatment
A = Airway Assess patient's ability to communicate Assess for signs of angio-oedema (swollen tongue/lips), obstruction (blood/secretions/broken teeth/tissue injury) secondary to upper airway/facial trauma Establish presence of added sounds and wheeze, stridor or gurgling noises Preparation for endotracheal or tracheostomy formation if facial trauma is present with compromised breathing	Identification of a compromised airway will prevent hypoxia and further cardio-respiratory complications. Presence of abnormal breathing sounds, cyanotic lips/tongue, difficulties in communication (incomplete/short sentences) may indicate a compromised airway. Trauma to the upper airway may lead to complete/partial airway obstruction (American College of Surgeons 2008)
B = Breathing Respiratory rate/depth/pattern Pulse oximetry – SpO_2	Assessment of respiratory status is important to establish O_2 demands and overall respiratory function – could identify potential trauma from collision. A patient in hypovolaemic shock having sustained multiple fractures will have increased respiratory demands to meet increased metabolic needs
Assess mechanics of breathing, i.e. bilateral/symmetrical chest wall rising Accessory muscle use Tracheal deviation Seesaw pattern	Paradoxical/abnormal breathing mechanics/tracheal deviation may indicate the presence of tension pneumothorax, haemothorax and flail chest
Evidence of duskiness/cyanosis in lips/tongue/ear lobes Chest X-ray (CXR)/CT scan	CXR/CT scan – to evaluate/confirm the impact of any trauma to the thoracic area. This may include identification of possible fractured ribs, pneumothorax/haemothorax
Arterial blood gases	Use of arterial blood gases (ABGs) when patient is critical can assess respiratory function, gaseous exchange PaO_2, $PaCO_2$, and pH values to inform intervention, i.e. whether patient requires intubation and ventilation or not
Auscultation	To identify air entry, the presence of any crackles or abnormal breathing sounds
Percussion	Examination of thoracic and abdominal resonance in the absence of radiological tests

can highlight the presence of respiratory complications or possible presence of bleeding (Resuscitation Council (UK) 2011)

C = Circulation
Temperature
Pulse rate (peripheral/central), rhythm and amplitude
Check pulse in limbs affected, i.e. pedal/tibial pulses
Check peripheral circulation for signs of deficit
Touch affected limbs to assess circulation/blood flow – compare with corresponding limb
Capillary refill time (CRT) (central)
Blood pressure
Remember
Monitor
Oxygen
Venous access
ECG

Haemodynamic assessment following fracture injury is essential. Trauma to bone tissue and associated supporting structures such as skeletal muscle and systemic circulation may compromise haemodynamic control and induce hypovolaemic shock. Complex, unstable and open fractures may lead to significant blood loss or ischaemia of tissue distal to fracture
Circulatory assessment may also identify physiological compensatory mechanisms in the presence of injury including BP alterations, increased pulse and delayed CRT
Record ECG and place on cardiac monitor – rule out cardiac arrhythmias induced by hypovolaemic loss and electrolyte derangement
IV access to facilitate fluid resuscitation

Obtain baseline bloods: full blood picture (FBP), urea and electrolytes, group and cross-match/hold

FBP significant to identify haemoglobin/platelets and white cell count in presence of hypovolaemia. Packed cells will be required in the presence of blood loss >20% of blood volume with no resolution of haemostatic control

Urinary catheterization

Identify renal function/perfusion in the presence of hypovolaemia

Central venous pressure (CVP) monitoring

CVP monitoring allows for an accurate assessment of haemodynamics if hypovolaemic shock is present (American College of Surgeons 2008)

D = Disability
AVPU
(Alert, responsive to Voice, Pain or Unresponsive)
GCS
Pupillary check – size, equality and reaction to light
Blood glucose measurement
Check for prescription/non-prescription drugs as a potential cause for accident

Neurological assessment is important to identify neurological deficit as a result of possible head injury
AVPU will indicate gross neurological damage only and is appropriate in the primary survey. GCS may wait until secondary assessment (Smith 2003)
To obtain baseline measurement and consider if further treatment is required
To establish if there is any impact on immediate treatment of the patient

(Continued overleaf)

Table 13.1 (*Continued*)

Assessment/investigations	Rationale
Pain assessment	Severe pain will impact on the physiological responses of the patient and will need to be addressed rapidly
E = Exposure Head-to-toe examination of patient for contusion, bleeding, laceration, swelling or deformity/shortening of affected limbs Assess loss of range of movements/mobility Serial X-rays of head, upper thorax, abdomen, and limbs. Posterior/anterior and lateral views reserved Wound assessment if present	Assessment of patient from head to toe will identify less obvious injury, lacerations/contusions/active bleeding X-rays are used as the primary tool to diagnose the type and location of fracture injury Abnormal rotation and loss of articulation between limbs can highlight the nature and extent of fracture trauma Differing views will identify the precise extent and severity of injury, examine fracture lines and demonstrate cortical continuity CT scan may be required for complex injuries with suspected internal organ damage Head-to-toe assessment may also identify the development of complications such as compartment syndrome (Dandy and Edwards 2009)

Clinical presentation

John's car left the road and rolled over several times before coming to a standstill. No other vehicles/casualties were involved. Patient was conscious when attended to by the paramedic crew and had complained of severe pain in his chest and legs. The patient arrives with a rigid collar, spinal board and cardiac monitor in place. High flow oxygen therapy and IV fluids have been established.

The patient is responsive on arrival; he is cold and clammy and has marked lacerations to the face. No active bleeding is noted elsewhere but his two lower legs are grossly oedematous, are mottled in appearance with faint pedal and tibial pulses recorded. The patient also presents with marked dyspnoea.

Radiological assessment highlights no evidence of cervical spine/brain damage; however, severe trauma is identified with contusion in right pleural lobe and multiple rib fractures with haemothorax to the left thoracic area. In addition, closed bilateral fractures of distal tibia and fibula of the left leg (oblique) and right (transverse) legs are noted.

Vital signs

Airway: gurgling and blood-stained sputum noted
Respiratory rate: 27 breaths per minute
Poor air entry on left thoracic area with loss of symmetry and use of accessory muscles
  noted
SpO$_2$: 83% (high flow O$_2$ 85% – non-rebreath mask)
Heart rate 115: beats per minute (sinus tachycardia)
Blood pressure: 80/40 mmHg
Temperature: 35.5°C
AVPU: A – alert
Glasgow Coma Scale: 15
Blood glucose: 5 mmol/L
Pain score: 10/10

---

3   **Explain John's clinical presentation in relation to the nature of his injuries. Discuss the underlying physiological changes that occur as a result of his injuries.**

A   Table 13.2 shows the clinical symptoms and the physiological changes.

Table 13.2 John's clinical symptoms and physiological changes

Clinical symptom	Cause	Physiological changes
Added sounds in airway, loss of symmetry in breathing mechanics	Thoracic contusion and haemothorax	Gurgling/blood-stained secretions in upper airway are indicative of internal bleeding within the thoracic area. Fractured bone tissue results in puncturing of pleural space and damage to blood vessels leading to lung collapse and loss of symmetry in thoracic expansion. The presence of air/fluid in the affected side will cause tracheal displacement away from collapsed pleura (Resuscitation Council (UK) 2011)
Hypotension ↑ CRT Cold/clammy Deranged neural functioning	Hypovolaemia secondary to blood loss in lower limbs Reduced cardiac output due to potential electrolyte imbalance as result of fluid loss	Circulating blood pressure falls due to lack of haemostatic control as a result of blood loss from the systemic circulation to interstitial/external spaces because of the vascular trauma at injury sites. The situation may persist, given the body's immediate inflammatory response with the release of histamine and other inflammatory mediators.
Tachycardia HR >100 beats per minute	Hypovolaemia Hypoxia	Volume loss will result in decreased peripheral blood flow as the vasomotor centre attempts to increase vascular resistance to maintain blood supply to essential organs (Flynn and McLeskey 2005)

(Continued overleaf)

Table 13.2 (*Continued*)

Clinical symptom	Cause	Physiological changes
Hypoxia ↑ RR ↓ SpO2	Haemothorax Haemorrhage	Compensatory mechanisms are initiated via stimulation of sympathetic nervous system (cardiac centre) by means of baroreceptors. This will initiate increased release of catecholamines which will increase heart rate and contractility in order to increase cardiac output
		Vascular loss and decreased blood volume will result in a reduction in haemoglobin and haematocrit, thus reducing the means of oxygen delivery to the cells. The presence of hypoxia will increase heart rate as the cardiac centre and heart attempt to meet metabolic requirements
		The development of a haemothorax decreases the lungs' functional ability, resulting in poor gaseous exchange and reduced O_2/CO_2 exchange. An increased level of CO_2 will stimulate the respiratory centre to augment rate and depth of breathing in an attempt to return the level to normal. Increased metabolic demands due to increased heart rate and the initiation of the inflammatory process at fracture site/s will demand greater O_2 for ATP production. Loss of red blood cells due to significant haemorrhage will decrease oxygen-carrying capacity of blood. In an attempt to compensate for these changes, the respiratory centre will stimulate increased respiratory effort (Dandy and Edwards 2009)
Pain 10/10	Trauma to nerve endings Inflammation	The immediate pain of a fracture is severe and usually caused by trauma to the periosteum and endosteum (double-layered connective tissue which contains nerves that penetrate to the inner structures of the bone). Subsequent pain may be produced by muscle spasm, over-riding of the fracture segments into skeletal muscle or soft tissue damage. At a biochemical level, release of prostaglandins (immediate) and later bradykinins released by mast cell breakdown induce pain by the stimulation of nerve endings (Crowther and Mourad 2010)

4   **Given the information provided, identify the patient's immediate priorities of care and nursing management of these. Provide a rationale for your interventions.**

A   Table 13.3 presents the priority of care and nursing management.

Table 13.3 Priority of care and nursing management

Problem	Intervention	Rationale
Potential of spinal injury following trauma	Assume cervical spine damage in all trauma cases Ensure spine is immobilized using appropriate aids Utilize appropriate moving and handling aids ensuring patient is 'log rolled' when undertaking therapeutic interventions	Immobilization of the spine including the cervical area is imperative at all times in the pre-hospital/in-hospital management of trauma until a complete assessment of the patient is undertaken. Secondary damage to the spine can lead to irreversible paralysis and loss of cardio-respiratory function (Aresco 2005)
Shortness of breath due to thoracic trauma and hypovolaemia	Seek expert help for advance airway management intervention and prepare appropriate airway adjuncts. Remove any blockages/secretions if present Monitor respiratory observations	Compromised airway/breathing will induce/prolong hypoxia leading to potential cardio-respiratory arrest Insertion of advanced airway will facilitate management of hypoxia Continuous respiratory observations will detect any deterioration/improvement in patient's condition
	Administer oxygen therapy 85% at 10–15 L per minute via non-rebreath mask	Given the limited oxygen diffusion due to the presence of chest trauma, high flow oxygen therapy is required to address increased metabolic demands. Aim to achieve oxygen saturations of between 94–98% (Resuscitation Council (UK) 2010)
	Position patient appropriately as condition permits	To facilitate increased lung expansion
	Prepare equipment for chest drain	Medical management of haemothorax requires removal of blood from pleural cavity so that normal function can be restored

(Continued overleaf)

Table 13.3 (*Continued*)

Problem	Intervention	Rationale
	Reserve/report findings from ABGs	Blood gases will identify derangement of respiratory function (changes in PaO_2, $PaCO_2$ and pH) and inform medical intervention (American College of Surgeons 2008)
	Restore blood volume with IV fluid administration	Prior to chest decompression with a chest drain, lost blood volume must be replaced to minimize the risk of haemodynamic decompensation and possible cardiac arrest
Hypotension as a result of bilateral fractures and thoracic trauma	Monitor cardiovascular observations	Close monitoring of cardiovascular observations is essential to assess haemodynamic state and to evaluate therapeutic interventions, e.g. fluid resuscitation
	Attach to cardiac monitor	Given the potential fluid loss cardiac monitoring is essential to evaluate the conduction and rhythm of the heart and assist in early identification of fatal arrhythmias
	Ensure insertion/management of 2 wide-bore cannula (14 g) Administer IV fluids – consider crystalloids, colloids, blood products	Fluid management must be fast and efficient to restore intravascular volume and maintain cardiac output (bolus challenge 500–1000 mL). Crystalloids are indicated as first-line fluid replacement with volumes 3–4 times that of estimated intravascular loss. Caution is required with excessive administration of crystalloids in cases with major chest trauma as it can contribute further to pulmonary congestion. Colloids (e.g. gelatins) can be used in relatively unrestricted volumes in fluid replacement. Once a patient has lost more than 30–40% of their blood volume, resuscitation with fluids possessing good O_2-carrying abilities is essential, i.e. packed red cells

	Reserve blood samples for full blood picture, urea and electrolytes, blood grouping	Baseline bloods will evaluate haemoglobin and haematocrit levels and establish Rhesus factor/blood type in the event of a packed cell transfusion being required (Flynn and McLeskey 2005)
Pain	Assess patient for pain using analogue pain intensity scale, identifying location(s), description, and associated symptoms	Establishing the intensity and characteristics of pain enables selection of appropriate analgesia and provides a baseline for evaluating the efficacy of interventions (Dougherty and Lister 2008)
	Administer analgesia as prescribed Evaluate and record discomfort and effectiveness of pain modifying techniques	Opioid administration is important once neurological assessment is established as it aids treatment of hypovolaemic shock by reducing catecholamine secretion. Avoid opioid administration in patients with head injury unless stable as this may distort the accuracy of neurological assessment and decrease consciousness level
	Avoid unnecessary movement of limbs	Immobilization of affected limbs reduces further trauma of nerve endings/damaged tissue (Whiteing 2008)
Monitoring of neurovascular function	Assess affected extremity for alterations in colour and temperature, capillary refill response and sensation Monitor pulses in lower extremities (pedal/tibial) Assess for deep throbbing unrelenting pain Inform medical staff in any change in symptoms as identified above	Venous congestion may cause cyanosis. Assessment of lower extremities will identify the extent of neurovascular injury and the development of complications Capillary refill measurement is accomplished by compression of the nail bed in the affected limb for 5 seconds. A rapid return capillary refill indicates good capillary perfusion Extensive bleeding into the musculature can result in compartment syndrome, and cause ischaemia in lower extremities Diminished pain and paraesthesia may indicate nerve damage (Dandy and Edwards 2009)

(Continued overleaf)

Table 13.3 (*Continued*)

Problem	Intervention	Rationale
Potential deterioration in neurological functioning as a result of trauma	Assess level of consciousness using AVPU (rapid assessment) (Alert, Responsive to Voice, Responsive to Pain, Unresponsive) or Glasgow Coma Scale Assess changes in size, equality, reactivity of patient's pupils Report deterioration if GCS falls by 2 points	Using AVPU will provide a rapid assessment of level of consciousness on initial assessment. A full assessment using GCS is advised as it provides greater specificity of patient's conscious level. Changes in size, equality and reactivity of the patient's pupils may provide diagnostic information in acute illness and highlight cerebral trauma or changes in intracranial pressure. If GCS is less than 9 or if it falls by 2 points, expert intervention maybe required. Reduction in level of consciousness is associated with potentially life-threatening conditions including airway obstruction (Smith 2003)

> John's condition has stabilized, a chest drain is inserted and an emergency transfer to theatre is arranged for internal fixation of his leg fractures. However, prior to transfer, he becomes unresponsive.

5 **Identify the potential causes of his deterioration and outline possible management strategies.**

A MANAGEMENT STRATEGIES

Summon expert help if not already available. Common complications may include:

- *Cardio-respiratory arrest*: Immediate ABC assessments, on confirmation of arrest summon crash team, commence cardiopulmonary resuscitation (CPR), and attach to defibrillator. Consider likely reversible causes – hypoxia, hypovolaemia, cardiac tamponade, pulmonary emboli.
- *Hypovolaemic shock (haemorrhage)*: This can result in neurological deterioration. Monitor GCS and cardiovascular and respiratory observations. Urgent fluid replacement is indicated. Immediate surgical intervention will be required once patient's condition permits.
- *Respiratory failure*: This may occur secondary to physical trauma to the lung tissue, over transfusion of crystalloids, poor chest movement or adult respiratory distress syndrome

(ARDS). In addition, short-term complications can include fat emboli (uncommon) which result in respiratory failure. Treatment involves oxygen therapy, advance airway management and urgent transfer to critical care facilities for ventilator support.

* *Undetected brain injury*: Reassess GCS. Assess for alterations in pupillary response/size, monitor cardiovascular/respiratory observations for signs of deterioration. Patient will require an urgent CT scan, with possible neurosurgical intervention.
* *Effects of analgesia*: Opioid administration will potentially suppress all key cardiac, respiratory and vasomotor centres in the medulla oblongata and may be exacerbated by deranged renal function. Consider antidote (naloxone) or other pain management strategies (Dandy and Edwards 2009; Hamblen and Simpson 2010; Resuscitation Council (UK) 2011).

Key points

* Rapid assessment of a trauma patient utilizing the ABCDE approach is required.
* Significant blood loss will accompany multiple traumas leading to hypovolaemic shock.
* Close monitoring of cardiovascular and neurovascular status is essential.

REFERENCES

American College of Surgeons (2008) *Advanced Trauma Life Support*, 8th edn. Washington, DC: American College of Surgeons.

Aresco, C.A. (2005) Trauma, in P. Morton, D. Fontaine, C. Hudak and B. Gallo (eds) *Critical Care Nursing: A Holistic Approach*, 8th edn. Philadelphia, PA: Lippincott Williams and Wilkins.

Crowther, C.L. and Mourad, L.A. (2010) Alterations in musculoskeletal function, in K.L. McCance and S.E. Heuther (eds) *Pathophysiology: The Biological Basis for Disease in Adults and Children*, 6th edn. St Louis, MO: Mosby.

Dandy, D.J. and Edwards, D.J. (2009) *Essential Orthopaedics and Trauma*, 5th edn. London: Churchill Livingstone.

Dougherty, L. and Lister, S. (eds) (2008) *The Royal Marsden Hospital Manual of Clinical Nursing Procedures*. Chichester: Wiley-Blackwell.

Flynn, M.B. and McLeskey, S. (2005) Shock, systemic inflammatory response syndrome, and multiple organ dysfunction syndrome, in P. Morton, D. Fontaine, C. Hudak and B. Gallo (eds) *Critical Care Nursing: A Holistic Approach*, 8th edn. Philadelphia, PA: Lippincott Williams and Wilkins.

Hamblen, D.L. and Simpson, A.H. (2010) *Adams's Outline of Orthopaedics*, 14th edn. London: Churchill Livingstone.

Resuscitation Council (UK) (2010) *Immediate Life Support*, 3rd edn. London: Resuscitation Council (UK).

Resuscitation Council (UK) (2011) *Advanced Life Support*, 6th edn. London: Resuscitation Council (UK).

Smith, G. (2003) *Acute Life-Threatening Events Recognition and Treatment (ALERT)*, 2nd edn. Portsmouth: University of Portsmouth.

Whiteing, N.L. (2008) Fractures: pathophysiology, treatment and nursing care, *Nursing Standard*, 23(2): 49–57.

PART 8
Multiple Interacting Systems

Shock: hypovolaemic
Karen Page

Case outline

Louise Cousins is a 36-year-old lady who had recently been diagnosed with acute myeloid leukaemia (AML). She is receiving an initial course of intensive induction chemotherapy in the haematology ward with the aim of producing remission in her condition. Although she was initially devastated by the diagnosis, she is responding to treatment with very good family support from her husband and parents. She also has a young daughter who is just 3 years old and she is really looking forward to spending time with her when she is discharged from hospital. She appeared to be tolerating the regime reasonably well although her appetite had decreased with the development of some diarrhoea in the past few days. This morning Louise spoke to the nurse who was preparing to administer her chemotherapy and described having had one episode of passing a small amount of fresh blood per rectum which seemed to her to be quite different to the episodes of diarrhoea which she had previously experienced.

---

1 **What is your initial course of action at this point?**

A It is vitally important to listen attentively to the patient describing her symptoms as one of the major complications of AML includes bleeding. AML results from a defect in the haematopoetic stem cell that differentiates into all myeloid cells: monocytes, granulocytes (neutrophils, basophils, eosinophils), erythrocytes and platelets. This may lead to the risk of patients developing bleeding disorders secondary to thrombocytopenia and altered coagulation due to malignant invasion of the bone marrow or bone marrow suppression resulting from the effects of chemotherapy. Moreover, gastrointestinal problems such as anorexia, nausea, vomiting, diarrhoea and severe mucositis may result from the infiltration of abnormal leukocytes into the abdominal organs and from the toxicity of the chemotherapy agents (Smeltzer et al. 2008). It is therefore vital to *seek urgent medical advice before proceeding with any further administration of chemotherapy agents* as the drug regime may be contributing to Louise's present symptoms. The nurse should advise the patient to notify the staff immediately if any further bleeding occurs so that a more rigorous appraisal of her symptoms can be undertaken. It is important for the nurse to note both the amount and colour of the bleed and whether this is bright red or dark-coloured as this may assist in establishing if the bleeding has originated from the upper or lower gastrointestinal tract. An urgent clinical assessment to obtain vital signs should also be completed to establish the patient's present condition. Given her diagnosis and her description of passing fresh blood, the frequency of recording her observations should be increased to monitor her condition closely. The use of an early warning system (EWS) will help to alert staff to any changes in her clinical observations in a timely fashion (NICE 2007).

Clinical observations are recorded as:

Temperature: 37.1°C
Blood pressure: 118/78 mmHg
Heart rate: 96 beats per minute
Respirations: 18 breaths per minute
Oxygen saturations: 97% on room air

Louise was not complaining of any pain and did not appear to be overtly unwell although she was quite anxious and agitated about this event. Routine blood samples including a group and cross-match were also obtained indicating Hb 9.8 g/dL (normal range 11.5–15.5 g/dL) and platelets 125 µL (normal range 150–400 µ/L).

---

2 **What further nursing action should be taken to support Louise during this time?**

A The nurse must ensure that in addition to the ongoing clinical monitoring of the patient, other essential aspects of patient management are addressed. Continued psychological support for the patient is required as she was anxious and concerned about the episode of bleeding which she had experienced. A cancer diagnosis and the subsequent treatment and uncertainty which a patient experiences can cause profound anxiety and distress to them (Skilbeck and Payne 2003). Good communication skills are vital in supporting this patient to cope with the additional stress of this episode. Nurses have considerable contact with patients and are therefore arguably well placed to assess and provide supportive and psychological care (Towers 2007). This should include the development of trusting and sensitive relationships and the provision of timely and accurate information to both the patient and their family. While it is difficult for the nurse to be specific as to the significance of the bleeding noted by the patient in this instance, it is important that the patient feels that her concerns are taken seriously to develop a trusting and supportive relationship. Providing brief explanations about the possible diagnostic and treatment procedures which may be required and providing information about their outcomes are often effective in reducing stress and anxiety, thus promoting the patient's physical and mental well-being.

Louise had two further small episodes of bleeding during the night of approximately 75–100 mL. Her clinical observations continued to be reasonably stable although changes were noted in her heart rate and respirations which had increased to 104 beats per minute and 22 respirations per minute respectively. She appeared pale and anxious and slept very little during the night. An urgent sigmoidoscopy was therefore performed the following morning in the ward. This did not show anything of significance but the decision was taken by the medical staff to prepare the patient for an oesophagogastroduodenoscopy (OGD) to determine if there was a potential cause for the bleeding higher up the gastrointestinal tract. However, before an OGD could be undertaken, Louise suddenly passed a substantial amount of fresh blood in one episode, approximately 1200 mL, leading to a rapid deterioration in her condition and the development of hypovolaemic shock.

A rapid ABC assessment of the patient at this point revealed the following information:

- *Airway*: Patent, however, as patient is now quite drowsy, she was positioned on her side to assist in maintaining a clear airway.
- *Breathing*: Respiratory rate 28 respirations per minute rapid and shallow, oxygen saturations dropping to 92% on 2 litres oxygen via nasal cannula. Patient was commenced on high flow oxygen @15 litres via a rebreath mask.
- *Circulation*: Pulse 134 beats per minute weak and thready, BP 82/50 mmHg, capillary refill > 4 seconds, colour pale, peripheries cold and clammy, temperature 37.4°C. Cardiac monitoring was commenced. Further bloods revealed Hb 5.3 g/dL and platelet count 75 µL. Blood gases were also obtained.

3   **Describe the physiological responses associated with the development of hypovolaemic shock and identify the progression of shock in this case.**

A   Shock describes a life-threatening condition which represents a major challenge to the homeostasis of body systems. It describes the clinical syndrome that occurs when acute circulatory failure with inadequate or inappropriately distributed perfusion results in failure to meet tissue metabolic demands, causing generalized cellular hypoxia (Porth 2007) (Figure 14.1). Hypovolaemic shock develops when blood volume is diminished to the point that an adequate cardiac output cannot be maintained. Haemorrhage is the most common cause of this loss although body fluid can be lost through other causes such as excessive vomiting, diarrhoea, dehydration or burns which can contribute to the development of shock.

The development of shock has been classified into three stages: compensatory, progressive and refractory or irreversible stage (Porth 2007).

- *Compensatory stage*: The initial compensatory stage of shock is characterized by the body's attempt to regain homeostasis and improve tissue perfusion (Garretson and Malberti 2007). The most immediate of the compensatory changes are the sympathetic mediated responses seen in Figure 14.2. Hormonal compensation initiated in response to low renal blood flow leads to activation of the renin–angiotensin–aldosterone system, which promotes vasoconstriction and water conservation in an effort to maintain intravascular volume and sufficient blood pressure to sustain tissue perfusion. The decrease in blood volume also stimulates the release of anti-diuretic hormone (ADH) which further increases vasoconstriction and water retention. The mechanism for ADH release is more sensitive to changes in serum osmolarity so a decrease of 10–15% in blood volume is a

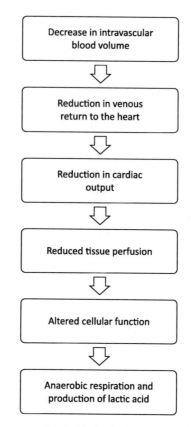

Figure 14.1 Physiological response associated with the development of hypovolaemic shock

strong stimulus for ADH secretion (Porth 2007). Although cellular changes are taking place, clinical signs and symptoms may be slight and difficult to detect at this early stage of shock, so it is vital to pay close attention to even the subtlest changes in vital signs such as an increase in respiratory or heart rates. This is evidenced by Louise whose observations remained relatively stable initially with only a slight rise in respiratory rate and pulse accompanied by anxiety, though the anxiety may also be increased by seeing the passage of fresh blood.

- *Progressive stage*: However, these compensatory mechanisms are finite and as fluid loss increases to more than 20% of blood volume, the body loses its ability to compensate for the loss of blood volume and changes in vital signs become obvious (Strickler 2010). The decrease in cellular perfusion results in metabolic acidosis, electrolyte imbalance and respiratory acidosis and other sequelae related to symptoms of progressive organ failure (Garretson and Malberti 2007). The clinical symptoms include severe hypotension, pallor, tachycardia and irregular cardiac rhythms, cool and clammy extremities and an altered level of consciousness. This has been demonstrated in Louise's case with the development of severe hypotension, which is an ominous sign that shock is progressing, and other changes to her clinical observations following the large blood loss experienced by the patient. The grave nature of her condition is now obvious.

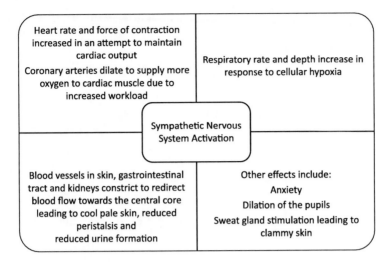

Figure 14.2 Neural compensation mediated via sympathetic nervous system

As Louise has continued to lose blood, her clinical symptoms have demonstrated the passage from compensated to the progressive stages of shock.

- *Refractory/irreversible stage*: If treatment is not instigated as a matter of urgency, then Louise will enter the refractory stage at which point the situation would become life-threatening with the occurrence of multiple organ damage and death (Porth 2007).

4   **Discuss the management of the patient following the development of hypovolaemic shock.**

A   Management of hypovolaemic shock, whatever the origin, is focused on resolving the under-lying cause, restoring fluid volume and blood pressure, thus reversing tissue hypoxia and preventing the vicious cycle of progressive organ damage (Figure 14.3). Consequently, as

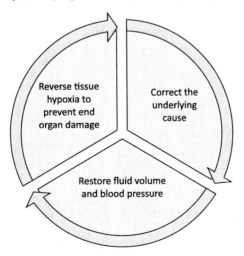

Figure 14.3 Management of hypovolaemic shock

Louise's condition is deteriorating rapidly at this point, it is important to stabilize this by immediate fluid resuscitation before attempting further investigations to establish the cause of the gastrointestinal bleeding.

Louise had a peripherally inserted central catheter (PICC) line in situ to facilitate delivery of her chemotherapy regime; however, two wide-bore peripheral cannulae were inserted to accommodate fluid resuscitation. 1 litre of sodium chloride 0.9% was prescribed stat. over 15 minutes. Four units of packed cells and two units of fresh frozen plasma were ordered for immediate transfusion by medical staff.

---

5 **Review the knowledge of blood groups and blood components which is required to support safe blood transfusion practice.**

A When a patient loses approximately 30–40% of their blood volume fluid, resuscitation should encompass not only crystalloid solutions but also blood components. The patient's haemoglobin level can be a useful indicator to trigger transfusion; however, clinical judgement and knowledge of patient's co-morbidities should also be taken into account. Louise already had a low haemoglobin and platelet count because of her existing AML. A unit of packed red cells contains the same amount of haemoglobin as a unit of whole blood and will therefore improve the oxygen-carrying capacity of the blood while helping to prevent excessive fluid overload. Many hospitals have a transfusion protocol for use in circumstances which dictate the administration of large amounts of blood and supplemental products (McClelland 2007). However, an understanding of the ABO compatibility of blood groups and antibodies is vital to support safe nursing practice in this area. This is summarized in Table 14.1.

Consequently, group O red cell units can be given to a patient of any ABO group in an urgent situation as the transfused cells have no A or B antigens to react with the recipient's antibodies. However, there is a risk of a haemolytic reaction if the patient has antibodies against other red cell antigens. This is most likely if the patient has had pregnancies or has previously been transfused with red cells with the RhD antibody being the most common of these (Watson and Hearnshaw 2010). In an emergency, the risk of reaction must therefore be balanced against the risk of undue delay in replacing blood loss as it is clear that any reaction would further exacerbate an already serious situation.

Table 14.1 ABO compatibility of blood and antibodies

Patient's ABO blood group	Patient's plasma contains	Red cell units that are compatible
O	Anti-A and-B antibodies	O
A	Anti-B antibodies	A and O
B	Anti-A antibodies	B and O
AB	Neither	A, B, AB and O

Source: McClelland (2007).

These naturally occurring antibodies are mainly IgM immunoglobulins which attack and rapidly destroy red cells. If red cells of an incompatible ABO group are transfused, the recipient's IgM immunoglobulins anti-A, anti-B and anti-AB bind to the transfused red cells. This activates the full complement pathway causing pores in the red cell membrane and destroying the transfused red cells in the circulation (intravascular haemolysis). Complement activation will also stimulate the release of cytokines such as tumour necrosis factor, interleukin-1 and interleukin-8 which stimulates degranulation of mast cells with the release of mediators such as histamine. This will lead to the activation of the inflammatory cascade, increased vascular permeability and hypotension which may in turn cause shock and renal failure (McClelland 2007).

Plasma is the fluid portion of the blood and can be processed into fresh frozen plasma (FFP) or cryoprecipitate. The same risks of ABO incompatibility therefore apply to transfusion of these blood components. During massive transfusion, regular monitoring of haemoglobin, platelet count, prothrombin time (PT), partial thromboplastin time (PTT) and fibrinogen levels should take place. Partial prothrombin time is a measure of the adequacy of the intrinsic and common pathways of the coagulation cascade. The body uses this cascade to produce blood clots to seal off injuries to blood vessels and tissues in an effort to prevent further blood loss and give the damaged areas time to heal. Along with measurement of prothrombin time (which evaluates the extrinsic and common pathways of the coagulation cascade), fibrinogen levels and platelet count can indicate the need for replacement of other blood components in acute blood loss (Creed and Spiers 2010).

6 **Consider the nursing role in the transfusion of blood components.**

A While it is a medical responsibility to prescribe blood components, the completion of a request form, taking a blood sample for pre-transfusion testing and administration of the blood component can be delegated to a nurse with appropriate training (RCN 2005). Therefore, the nurse has a responsibility to adhere to the local trust/hospital guidelines to ensure patient safety in all aspects of treatment, as failure to do so may result in significant patient harm. Even in an emergency situation such as is present in this case, it is of vital importance that policies and procedures related to blood transfusion are strictly adhered to by all those involved in Louise's care.

Think: principles of administration of blood and blood products

1   Every patient who receives a transfusion of blood or blood products should be given a full explanation about proposed treatment. However, in the case of a patient who receives an urgent blood transfusion to treat an acute bleeding episode, this must necessarily be brief and concise. If the patient is unconscious or unable to give consent, the decision to transfuse blood to the patient will be taken by the medical staff in the best interests of the patient.

2   The transfusion should begin as soon as the blood has arrived in the clinical area. Rapid infusion may be required, e.g. a unit over 5–10 minutes to manage a major haemorrhage.

3   The nurse should record baseline observations of temperature, pulse, blood pressure and respiratory rate before starting the transfusion of each unit of blood or blood component.

4 Positive patient identification is essential to avoid errors. All the relevant checks of patient identification *must* be carried out as per hospital policy at the bedside and whenever possible involving the patient. The bedside check is the last point at which any previous errors can be detected so it is vital that this is performed correctly (RCN 2005; 2010).

5 Ensure the patient is closely observed for any adverse reactions such as shivering, flushing, pain or shortness of breath.

6 Monitor the patient's temperature, pulse and other observations 15 minutes after beginning the transfusion of each unit and record as per hospital/trust policy. Severe reactions are most likely to occur in the first 15 minutes of transfusions (Watson and Hearnshaw 2010).

7 Observations must be carried out and recorded for each separate unit of blood. Infusion rates depend on the individual situation and must be specified by the medical staff. Ensure that the flow rate is adjusted to deliver the infusion over the prescribed time period.

8 Blood components must be transfused through a blood administration set with an integral mesh filter (170–200 μm pore size) (McClelland 2007).

9 Only use an infusion pump if they are certified as suitable for blood components by the manufacturer. Rapid infusion devices may be used if large volumes of blood are to be transfused swiftly. These usually incorporate a blood warming device.

10 Hypothermia impairs blood clotting. Blood warmers can be used for blood components provided that they are specifically designed for that purpose and include a visible thermometer and audible alarm (Bishop 2008; Hanvey 2008). *Never improvise by warming blood components in hot water, in a microwave or on a radiator* (McClelland 2007; RCN 2010).

11 Fresh frozen plasma should usually be transfused within 30 minutes as the efficacy of coagulation factors reduces once thawed.

12 Record the volume of blood and other fluids transfused in addition to the urinary and other output measures accurately on the fluid balance chart to assist in evaluating the adequacy of fluid replacement.

7 Who else must be informed of these developments in the patient's condition?

A Relatives should always be informed of any change in a patient's condition as a matter of urgency. Often there is little time to prepare relatives for a critical intervention or sudden change in a patient's condition. As nurses spend more time forming relationships with patients and their relatives, they are in a better position than medical staff to support relatives at critical times. Because shock syndromes can develop very quickly, families may be overwhelmed and frightened. They may be reluctant to ask questions or seek information for fear that they may be in the way or take away from the attention given to the patient. The nurse should be aware of this and ensure that the family is kept fully informed about the patient's status (Smeltzer et al. 2008).

Louise's condition continued to deteriorate with further episodes of bleeding and a further drop in blood pressure despite fluid resuscitation measures. The critical care outreach team, in consultation with the ward staff, therefore decided to move the patient to the Intensive Care Unit (ICU). During this time Louise was given continuous infusions of packed cells and crystalloids to support her cardiovascular system. In ICU she was placed on a ventilator, had an arterial line and central venous catheter inserted to monitor her condition closely and required inotrope support to maintain her blood pressure. When her condition stabilized, she was investigated to determine the cause of bleeding. This demonstrated extensive areas of ulceration lining the gastrointestinal tract, as a result of mucositis following chemotherapy.

Key points

- Knowledge of disease processes and side effects of drug therapy is crucial.
- Treatment of shock involves adequate and timely fluid resuscitation to support the cardiac output.
- Adherence to patient safety checks is vital even in emergency situations.

REFERENCES

Bishop, L. (2008) Blood transfusion therapy, in L. Dougherty and J. Lamb (eds) *Intravenous Therapy in Nursing Practice*. Oxford: Blackwell Publishing.

Creed, F. and Spiers, C (2010) *Care of the Acutely Ill Adult: An Essential Guide for Nurses*. Oxford: Oxford University Press.

Garretson, S. and Malberti, S. (2007) Understanding hypovolaemic, cardiogenic and septic shock, *Nursing Standard*, 50(21): 46–55.

Hanvey, N. (2008) Transfusion of blood and blood products, in L. Dougherty and S. Lister (eds) *The Royal Marsden Hospital Manual of Clinical Nursing Procedures*, 7th edn. Oxford: Blackwell Publishing.

McClelland, D.B.L. (2007) *Handbook of Transfusion Medicine*, 4th edn, United Kingdom Blood Services. London: The Stationery Office.

NICE (National Institute for Clinical Excellence) (2007) *Acutely Ill Patients in Hospital: Recognition and Response to Acute Illness of Adults in Hospital*. London: HMSO.

Porth, C.M. (2007) *Essentials of Pathophysiology: Concepts of Altered Health Status*, 2nd edn. Philadelphia, PA: Lippincott Williams and Wilkins.

RCN (Royal College of Nursing) (2005) *Right Blood, Right Patient, Right Time: RCN Guidance for Improving Transfusion Practice*. London: RCN.

RCN (Royal College of Nursing) (2010) *Standards for Infusion Therapy*, 3rd edn. London: RCN.

Skilbeck, J. and Payne, S. (2003) Emotional support and the role of clinical nurse specialists in palliative care, *Journal of Advanced Nursing*, 43(5): 521–30.

Smeltzer, S.C., Bare, B.G., Hinkle, J.L. and Cheever, K.H (2008) *Brunner and Suddarth's Textbook of Medical-Surgical Nursing*, 11th edn. Philadelphia, PA: Lippincott Williams and Wilkins.

Strickler, J. (2010) Traumatic hypovolemic shock: halt the downward spiral, *Nursing 2010* October: 34–9.

Towers, R. (2007) Providing psychological support for patients with cancer, *Nursing Standard*, 22(12): 50–7.

Watson, D. and Hearnshaw, K. (2010) Understanding blood groups and transfusion in nursing practice, *Nursing Standard*, 24(30): 41–8.

Shock: sepsis
Aidín McKinney

Case outline

Mrs Muriel Brown is a 48-year-old lady who has been admitted to A&E with a chesty cough and shortness of breath. She attended her G P approximately 5 days ago and was being treated for a suspected chest infection. Today her condition has deteriorated. She visited her G P again who was concerned that her condition appeared to have worsened and has advised her that she requires a chest X-ray and hospital treatment. On arrival at the A&E unit, her observations are as follows:

Temperature: 38.2°C
Pulse: 105 beats per minute
Blood pressure: 138/60 mm Hg
Respiratory rate: 22 breaths per minute
Oxygen saturations: 93%
White cell count: 9,000x 10^9/L.

---

1 **Reflect on the scenario above and consider how Muriel's signs and symptoms may be indicative of sepsis.**

A The scenario above indicates that Muriel has sepsis as she has a known or suspected infection, which is accompanied by two or more of the systemic inflammatory response syndrome (SIRS) criteria. The SIRS criteria have been identified as:

- High or low temperature >38°C or <36°C
- Heart rate >90 beats per minute
- Respiratory rate >20 breaths per minute or $PaCO_2$ (partial pressure of arterial carbon dioxide) <4.3 kPa
- High or low white blood cell count >12,000 or <4000x 10^9/L (Dellinger et al. 2004).

From Muriel's observations, it is apparent that she meets three of the SIRS criteria, i.e. her temperature is higher than 38°C, her heart rate is greater than 90 beats per minute, and her respiratory rate is greater than 20.

Unfortunately it is not always identified at an early enough stage that these symptoms indicate that the patient has sepsis. Sepsis tends to be a word that is commonly used in clinical practice; however, there has been a general lack of consensus about how it should be defined. Unfortunately it has tended to be the case that all too often a patient was only considered to have sepsis if their temperature was above 38.5°C and their white cell count was raised. However, as the above criteria demonstrate, these are not the only two SIRS criteria that are indicative of sepsis. Furthermore, it is worth noting that while a high temperature and a high white cell count are commonly associated with sepsis, it is not as common for nurses to also consider a diagnosis of sepsis based on a low temperature or a low white cell count (Robson et al. 2006). This is a useful point to emphasize in the hope that a diagnosis of sepsis will be recognized at the earliest possible stage (Robson and Newell 2005). Unfortunately, it would appear that a diagnosis of sepsis is frequently missed (Poeze et al. 2004; Robson et al. 2006). Increased awareness of the signs and symptoms of sepsis, however, is essential so that early and aggressive treatment is initiated as soon as possible to help prevent the condition deteriorating further.

2 **What simple interventions can or should be done when sepsis is suspected? Provide a rationale for these.**

A To appropriately diagnose and treat patients, a full set of relevant diagnostic tests must be undertaken. This is particularly important in patients who are suspected of having sepsis due to the many possible origins of the infection. It is therefore important to consider the clinical features and history of each patient as this should help direct the nurse or doctor to more specifically undertake key investigations. For example, in Muriel's case, with her history of having a chesty cough and shortness of breath, it would seem appropriate to consider obtaining a sputum sample and carrying out a chest X-ray. In patients with sepsis, it is essential that the underlying cause of the infection, and its extent must be ascertained as soon as possible if the source is to be treated effectively and a positive patient outcome is maximized (Pomeroy 2009).

Biochemistry samples are also important to provide an insight into the degree of sepsis in patients. This should include monitoring for an increase in the blood concentration of C-reactive protein and also a raised OR a low white cell count as these all provide information as to the degree of infection.

Regular monitoring of basic observations are particularly useful as these should readily point to clear signs of deterioration, particularly if used in conjunction with early warning score (EWS) charts. In particular, respiratory rate is now recognized as one of the earliest and most sensitive indicators of deterioration and indeed is one of the recognized SIRS criteria for sepsis, yet, unfortunately, this observation continues to be poorly performed (Hogan 2006). Indeed, concerns about the failure to recognize signs of deterioration at an early enough stage have led the National Institute for Health and Clinical Excellence to issue guidelines (NICE 2007) which recommend that carrying out a set of observations should include the following parameters as a minimum: respiratory rate, pulse, blood pressure, temperature, level of consciousness and that an EWS should be calculated for each set of observations.

At this point, results from the sputum sample may indicate a chest infection. If so, it is imperative that the appropriate antibiotics are commenced as soon as possible, thus hopefully preventing Muriel from becoming acutely ill. A diagnosis of sepsis is not in itself an indication of being acutely ill; however, it should be a warning of the potential to become so. Sepsis is a continuum, from a simple uncomplicated infection to a diagnosis of severe sepsis where there is an infection associated with compromised organ function and therefore an increased risk of becoming very seriously unwell (Robson and Daniels 2008).

Following initial investigations, Muriel is admitted to a medical ward. Later on that evening the staff nurse notices a deterioration in her condition. Her observations now indicate:

Temperature: 38.5°C
Pulse: 118 beats per minute
Blood pressure: 87/56 mmHg
Respiratory rate: 24 breaths per minute
Oxygen saturations: 89%
White cell count: 22,000x10^9/L
Urine output: approximately 20 mL per hour for the past 2 hours consecutively.

---

3 **What could have contributed to the deterioration in Muriel's condition?**

A Muriel could currently be diagnosed as having severe sepsis since she has fulfilled the criteria of sepsis as noted earlier, which is now associated with organ dysfunction. The criteria for associated organ dysfunction are:

- Hypotension: systolic blood pressure <90 mmHg, mean arterial pressure (MAP) <65 mmHg, or a reduction of >40 mmHg from the patient's usual reading.
- Lactate >4 mmol/L.
- Altered mental state.
- Hyperglycaemia in the absence of diabetes.
- Hypoxaemia, oxygen saturations ≤93%.
- Urine output <0.5 mL/kg/hr and/or a raised urea or creatinine.
- Coagulopathy, INR >1.5 (Peel 2008).

It is evident that in Muriel's case, she has at least three of the criteria associated with organ dysfunction as she is hypotensive (BP is 87/56 mmHg), she is hypoxic (oxygen saturations are 89%), and urine output is reduced (20 mL per hour for the past 2 hours consecutively).

The Surviving Sepsis Campaign guidelines for managing severe sepsis (Dellinger et al. 2004) state that it is essential to recognize the diagnosis of severe sepsis early and to treat aggressively if more patients are to survive.

4 **Identify the signs and symptoms that Muriel is or may be experiencing as a result of severe sepsis and explain these in relation to the underlying pathophysiology.**

A Table 15.1 shows the signs and symptoms of severe sepsis and their pathophysiology.

Table 15.1 Signs and symptoms of severe sepsis and their pathophysiology

Signs and symptoms	Pathophysiology
Feeling hot and flushed	When there is an invasion of foreign material such as bacteria, an inflammatory response is triggered. The first stage in the inflammatory response results in the release of various inflammatory mediators into the circulation, such as histamine, cytokines, prostaglandins and interleukins (Robson and Newell 2005). These promote an increase in blood flow to the site of the injury through vasodilation. This results in the classic signs of vasodilation being observed and the patient can appear red (erythema) and feel hot and flushed (Steen, 2009)
Hypotension	The release of the inflammatory mediators, which result in massive vasodilation also cause hypotension in severe sepsis. This is further compounded by the increased permeability that occurs in the capillaries also as a result of the release of inflammatory mediators, which allows fluid to leak out from the circulation into the interstitial space (Robson and Daniels 2008). This can result in a major loss of volume from the core circulation. The consequence of this can be significant organ dysfunction. An initial rise in diastolic pressure, followed by a drop in blood pressure and alterations in temperature, point towards late signs of a lack of oxygen supply to the tissues (Morton and Fontaine 2009). However, it is also important to point out that, unlike hypovolaemic shock secondary to haemorrhage, or cardiogenic shock that occurs following an acute myocardial infarction, hypotension is not always present in severe sepsis. Nevertheless it is important to be aware that although the patient may not be showing signs of hypotension, the delivery of oxygen to their tissues and organs may still be impaired. This phenomenon is known as 'cryptic shock' (Robson and Daniels 2008)
Rapid, bounding pulse	Due to the profound systemic vasodilation that occurs in severe sepsis, the venous return and stroke volume (the amount of blood ejected by the ventricle during contraction) fall, resulting in a reduction in cardiac output. To compensate, the body raises the heart rate and releases adrenaline in order to improve cardiac output. This results in an increased heart rate and bounding pulse (Steen 2009)
Hyperglycaemia	Hyperglycaemia is frequent in sepsis even in patients who do not have a history of diabetes or impaired glucose metabolism. Severe sepsis is associated with a hypermetabolic stress response and affects protein, lipid and carbohydrate metabolism throughout the body resulting in hyperglycaemia (Yu et al. 2003). It is also a consequence of the inflammatory response. Excess cytokine production results in insulin resistance and therefore also contributes to a rise in blood sugar levels (Gornik et al. 2010)

Raised blood lactate level	Physiological changes to the cardiovascular system that occur in severe sepsis as outlined above can cause a reduction in oxygen supply to cells, resulting from tissue hypoperfusion. This results in a change from aerobic to anaerobic cellular respiration or metabolism, which produces lactic acid (Robson and Newell 2005). A patient who has a lactate level greater than 4 mmol/L should be considered as having severe sepsis even if the blood pressure is within the normal range (Robson and Newell 2005)
Decreased urine output	The combined effect of a loss of venous return and a loss of circulating blood volume results in a significant reduction in cardiac output. Consequently, blood flow to the kidneys is reduced. The body initially compensates by activating the rennin–angiotensin–aldosterone system, increasing vascular tone and conserving fluid by reducing urine output. Eventually, however, if cardiac output does not improve, the compensatory mechanisms will fail and renal failure can ensue (Steen 2009)
Reduced oxygen saturations	The reduction in cardiac output and blood flow results in an inadequate oxygen supply to the tissues resulting in hypoxia (Steen 2009)
Altered mental state	Hypoxia can lead to confusion as a result of the brain being inadequately perfused (Robson and Newell 2005)
Coagulopathy	The coagulation system also becomes activated in severe sepsis and small blood clots or microthrombi form in the small blood vessels. These thrombi can interfere with blood flow to the organs and tissues, further contributing to organ failure (Robson and Newell 2005). Normally the body will attempt to break down any blood clots by fibrinolysis. However, in severe sepsis, fibrinolysis is inhibited by the release of plasminogen-activator inhibitor (PAI) thereby preventing the breakdown of microthrombi. Furthermore, the inflammatory and procoagulation response is very persistent, to the extent that the body is unable to maintain homeostasis (Robson and Newell, 2005)

5 **What interventions need to be considered once it has been identified that Muriel has signs and symptoms of severe sepsis? Consider the nurse's role in relation to these.**

A Once severe sepsis is identified, the Surviving Sepsis Campaign recommends that the Sepsis Six care bundle is implemented within the first six hours (Dellinger et al. 2008). A care bundle is a collection of interventions, each of which is based on identified best knowledge or practice, and collectively when carried out is said to produce a better outcome for the patient and improve survival (Steen 2009). Many of the interventions do not require specialized staff or equipment and can easily be instigated by staff nurses and junior doctors working in general wards. These six simple interventions are called the 'Sepsis Six' and are the first steps towards completing the Surviving Sepsis Campaign's resuscitation bundle. These are:

1 *Administer 85–100% oxygen therapy*: All patients identified as having severe sepsis should receive high flow oxygen therapy via a non-rebreath mask. The metabolic demands for oxygen are massively increased in sepsis and this type of mask delivers the closest to 100% oxygen that can be achieved with a face mask. It is important for the nurse to recognize that high flow oxygen will lead to drying of the patient's mouth and tracheal mucosa and therefore, if prolonged, humidified oxygen should be considered if it is available (Robson and Daniels 2008).

2 *IV fluid therapy*: Patients with severe sepsis will require IV fluid therapy to restore circulating volume that was lost from the 'leaky' capillaries. Fluid resuscitation should follow the fluid challenge principle. Dellinger et al. (2008) recommend giving boluses of 500–1000 mL of a crystalloid solution such as Hartmann's solution or 30–500 mL of colloid over 30 minutes, with a more rapid rate if there are significant signs of hypoperfusion. It is the nurse's role to monitor closely for any response to the fluid challenge, including an improvement in blood pressure and/or urine output. It is also important to monitor for signs of cardiac insufficiency, such as acute shortness of breath as, for example, may occur if the patient had a history of heart failure. If so, the volume of fluid needs to be reduced or administered more cautiously (Steen 2009).

3 *Ensure blood cultures are obtained*: It is important that blood cultures are taken before the patient is commenced on antibiotic therapy in order to obtain the best chance of isolating the causative organism. It is vital that these are taken using strict aseptic technique from a peripheral vein and if the patient has central line or peripheral cannula in situ, then blood cultures should be taken from these also (Robson and Daniels 2008).

4 *IV antibiotics*: After blood cultures are taken, broad spectrum antibiotics must be given intravenously as soon as possible, preferably within one hour of recognition of severe sepsis. This is important since each hour of delay is associated with a significant increase in mortality (Steen 2009).

5 *Insert catheter and monitor urine output*: Urinary output is a sensitive measure of blood flow to the kidneys but can also serve as an indication of blood flow to organs in general. The insertion of a urinary catheter with the commencement of hourly measurement of urine output is required to accurately measure urine output in patients. This should ideally be maintained at >0.5 mL/kg/hour (Steen 2009).

6 *Measure serum lactate and haemoglobin levels*: Raised lactate levels have been shown to be of vital prognostic importance in the septic patient. A lactate level of >4 mmol/L in the presence of severe sepsis gives a diagnosis of septic shock, regardless of the patient's blood pressure. Lactate levels can be easily measured from an arterial blood gas sample or by sending an urgent venous sample to the laboratory. If raised above 4 mmol/L, treatment for septic shock should commence as soon as possible. Haemogloblin levels are also useful to obtain, as, if low, the amount of oxygen carried to tissues and organs is reduced. Thus, if the haemoglobin level is less than 7 g/dL, it is recommended that a blood transfusion is commenced (Robson and Daniels 2008; Steen 2009).

Muriel is given a fluid challenge of 1 litre of Hartmann's solution over 30 minutes; however, her blood pressure remains low and she has not had any urinary response.

6   **What does the ward nurse now need to consider?**

A   Further fluid challenges will need to be considered. Fluid resuscitation is a key aspect in the treatment of a patient with severe sepsis. Indeed, it has been estimated that as much as 6–10 litres of fluid may have to be administered in the first 24 hours (Peel 2008). However, if hypotension or raised lactate does not improve with adequate fluid resuscitation, the patient may now be considered as having septic shock (Robson and Newell 2005). At this stage, the patient is critically ill and requires transfer to a High Dependency Unit (HDU) or Intensive Care Unit (ICU) for more invasive monitoring and aggressive therapy. This will include the need for insertion of a central venous catheter to more closely monitor responses to fluid challenges. Insertion of a central line will also allow more invasive treatment of ongoing hypotension with vasopressors, such as noradrenaline (Peel 2008). Other treatments that will be considered when the patient is transferred to a critical care area include ensuring glucose control with intravenous insulin therapy and the administration of corticosteroid therapy. Although the evidence for corticosteroid therapy has not been proven, there is some evidence to suggest that the use of corticosteroids may reverse the symptoms of shock. Lung protective strategies, probably through the use of ventilation, may also need to be employed (Steen 2009). The ward nurse therefore needs to be aware of the significance of a failure to respond to fluid challenges in order to summon appropriate help early, liaise with the relevant critical care outreach team and help to organize and facilitate the safe transfer of the patient.

Key points

- Sepsis is a life-threatening medical emergency.
- Increased awareness of the signs and symptoms of sepsis is essential so that early and aggressive treatment is initiated as soon as possible.
- Once severe sepsis is identified, the Surviving Sepsis Campaign recommends that the Sepsis Six care bundle is implemented within the first six hours.

REFERENCES

Dellinger, R.P., Carlet, J.M., Masur, H. et al. (2004) Surviving Sepsis Campaign guidelines for management of severe sepsis and septic shock, *Critical Care Medicine*, 32(3): 858–73.

Dellinger, R.P., Levy, M.M., Carlet, J.M., et al. (2008) Surviving Sepsis Campaign: international guidelines for management of severe sepsis and septic shock, *Critical Care Medicine*, 36(1): 296–327.

Gornik, I., Vujaklija, A., Lukic, E., Madzarac, G. and Gaspavrovic, V. (2010) Hyperglycaemia in sepsis is a risk factor for development of type II diabetes. *Journal of Critical Care*, 25(2): 263–9.

Hogan, J. (2006) Why don't nurses monitor the respiratory rates of patients? *British Journal of Nursing*, 15(9): 489–92.

Morton, P.G. and Fontaine, D. K. (2009) *Critical Care Nursing: A Holistic Approach*, 9th edn. Philadelphia, PA: Lippincott, Williams and Wilkins.

NICE (National Institute for Health and Clinical Excellence) (2007) *Acutely Ill Patients in Hospital: Recognition of and Response to Acute Illness in Adults in Hospital*. London: NICE.

Peel, M. (2008) Care bundles: resuscitation of patients with severe sepsis, *Nursing Standard*, 23(11): 41–6.

Poeze, M., Ramsay, G., Gerlach, H., Rubulotta, F. and Levy, M. (2004) An international sepsis survey: a study of doctors' knowledge and perception about sepsis, *Critical Care*, 8(6): 409–13.

Pomeroy, M. (2009) A patient with sepsis: an evaluation of care, *Emergency Nurse*, 17(2): 12–17.

Robson, W., Beavis, S. and Spittle, N. (2006) An audit of ward nurses' knowledge of sepsis, *Nursing in Critical Care*, 12(2): 86–92.

Robson, W. and Daniels, R. (2008) The Sepsis Six: helping patients to survive sepsis, *British Journal of Nursing* 17(1): 16–21.

Robson, W. and Newell, J. (2005) Assessing, treating and managing patients with sepsis, *Nursing Standard*, 19(50): 56–64.

Steen, C. (2009) Developments in the management of patients with sepsis, *Nursing Standard*, 23(48): 48–55.

Yu, W., Li, W., Li, N. and Li, J. (2003) Influence of acute hyperglycaemia in human sepsis on inflammatory cytokine and counterregulator, *World Journal of Gastroenterology*, 9(8): 1824–7.

Shock: anaphylactic
Aidín McKinney

Case outline

Christine is a 17-year-old student who has been complaining of a very sore throat for the past four days. Despite taking cold and flu medications at home, she feels that her symptoms are getting worse. She arranges an appointment with her GP. During her assessment, it was identified that Christine had severe tonsillitis. Her throat was red and inflamed and Christine was complaining of feeling very unwell and finding it difficult and painful to swallow. In addition, she had a temperature of 38.2°C. In view of her symptoms, her GP decided to refer her to the ear, nose and throat (ENT) department of the local hospital where she was admitted with a quinsy infection. She has a history of asthma and mild panic attacks but no other significant medical history. She also has no known drug allergies. Shortly after admission to the ward she was commenced on an IV infusion of amoxicillin 1 g. Within five minutes of the infusion commencing, she developed a red rash on her face and upper chest. She also appeared to be extremely anxious and was pointing to her throat which was swollen. She was finding it very difficult to breathe and on closer examination, an audible wheeze could be heard. The staff nurse present is concerned and calls for help. Vital signs are recorded and are as follows:

Respiratory rate: 32 breaths per minute
BP: 95/56 mmHg
Heart rate: 115 beats per minute

---

1 Discuss how you would assess Christine in order to confirm that she has developed an anaphylactic reaction.

A Anaphylaxis is an acute, severe and life-threatening allergic reaction. As such, it is vital that nurses appreciate that this is an acute emergency situation and recognize the signs early so that appropriate prompt treatment can be instigated as soon as possible. Otherwise there is a high possibility that their patient could die within minutes (East 2010).

The first step that should be taken in order to confirm that Christine has developed an anaphylactic reaction must be carrying out a quick assessment using the ABCDE approach (Resuscitation Council (UK) 2008) (Table 16.1).

Table 16.1 The ABCDE procedure in the case of anaphylaxis

ABCDE	Symptoms
A = Airway	From the scenario above, it is apparent that Christine has an airway problem. There is evident swelling around her throat. She also appears to be finding it difficult to speak as she only feels capable of pointing to her throat. There is also an audible wheeze present which suggests some degree of airway obstruction
B = Breathing	The scenario indicates that Christine is finding it difficult to breathe. Her respiratory rate is increased at 32 respirations per minute and she is wheezing. She may also be using her accessory muscles and may become tired or cyanosed
C = Circulation	There is evidence of some circulatory problems as noted by the increased pulse rate (tachycardia) and low blood pressure (hypotension). Christine may also be feeling faint or dizzy at this point and may look pale and feel clammy to touch
D = Disability	At this stage, using the AVPU scale it is apparent that Christine is alert and conscious
E = Exposure	Christine has a red rash on her face and upper chest. As identified by the Resuscitation Council (UK) (2008) skin changes such as a patchy or generalized rash can often be one of the first features of a reaction and are present in over 80% of anaphylactic reactions

Source: Resuscitation Council (UK) (2008).

According to the Resuscitation Council (UK) (2008), the diagnosis of anaphylaxis is likely when all of the following criteria are met (Figure 16.1):

- an acute or sudden onset of symptoms;
- life-threatening airway and/or breathing and/or circulation problems;
- and usually skin changes, such as redness, flushing and urticaria.

From the scenario above, it is evident that Christine meets the Resuscitation Council (UK) (2008) guidelines for having developed an anaphylactic reaction. She developed an acute onset of illness within five minutes of receiving intravenous amoxicillin. She has a life-threatening airway problem as there is obvious swelling around her throat. Her breathing is also compromised as evident from the fast respiratory rate and wheeze. She also has a circulation problem which can be identified from the low blood pressure. In addition, skin changes are apparent from the red rash on her face and upper chest. A diagnosis of an anaphylactic reaction can therefore be confirmed.

2 **How would you distinguish this from a panic attack?**

A It has been acknowledged that there can be confusion between the diagnosis of an anaphylactic reaction and panic attacks (Resuscitation Council (UK) 2008). Given that Christine has a history of experiencing mild panic attacks, it is therefore of particular importance to

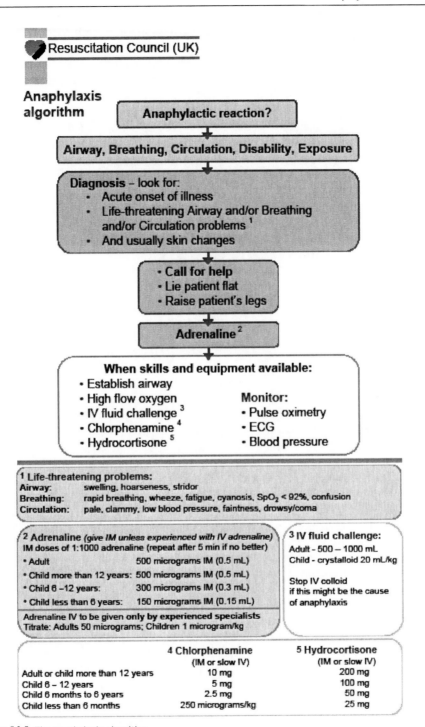

Figure 16.1 The anaphylaxis algorithm

Source: Resuscitation Council (UK) (2008).

consider how to differentiate between the two. The sense of impending doom or profound anxiety and shortness of breath are symptoms that resemble both anaphylaxis and panic attacks. The development of flushing or blotchy skin that sometimes accompanies acute anxiety can also give the appearance of a rash, further adding to the diagnostic difficulty. However, during a panic attack a patient is more likely to be hypertensive rather than hypotensive as occurs in the case of anaphylaxis. The absence of any signs of swelling around the airway are further distinguishing features that will point to a diagnosis of a panic attack as opposed to an anaphylactic reaction (Resuscitation Council (UK) 2008; East 2010). This highlights that the diagnosis of anaphylaxis may not always be immediately obvious and thus reinforces the importance of carrying out a full systematic ABCDE assessment in order to clearly ensure that an anaphylactic reaction is correctly identified.

3   **What is the immediate care that needs to be given to this patient?**

A   It is evident from the scenario that this patient is very seriously unwell. It is vital that this is recognized as soon as possible and, in the case of an anaphylactic reaction, that the initial management involves stopping the administration of the causative agent (in this case the IV infusion of amoxicillin) and that help is immediately called for (Linton and Watson 2010). The patient then needs to be assessed (or reassessed) and treatments commenced based on the ABCDE approach.

Ensuring that the patient has a clear airway is obviously a key priority. Christine appears to have some degree of airway obstruction as there is notable swelling around her throat, an audible wheeze is present and she is having difficulty breathing. Administration of high flow oxygen 15 litres/minute via a non-rebreath mask with an oxygen reservoir bag is a key first priority and will reduce the likelihood of hypoxia (Jevon 2010). An early request for senior help is also vital at this stage. The presence of angio-oedema suggests possible pending airway obstruction and thus consideration must be given to the possibility of Christine requiring early intubation of the airway as the procedure is likely to become more difficult as the oedema progresses (Linton and Watson 2010). Consideration of the patient's position at this stage is also important. Christine has some degree of hypotension and while the supine position may be helpful for this, it would be clearly unhelpful in respiratory distress (Jevon 2010). A semi-upright position may therefore be the best compromise for Christine at this point. Adrenaline should also be administered IM as soon as possible if there are clinical signs of shock or airway swelling, as is apparent in this scenario. Indeed, the earlier that this is given, the better the clinical outcome is likely to be (Royal College of Physicians 2009). The recommended dose in adults is 500 mcg IM (0.5 mL of 1:1000 solution) and this can be repeated after five minutes if there is no clinical improvement (Resuscitation Council (UK) 2008). The effects of adrenaline in treating anaphylaxis will be considered in more detail below. The patient's condition should be constantly monitored during this stage and observed for any signs of improvement or indeed deterioration and therefore oxygen saturations, blood pressure and electrocardiogram (ECG) monitoring should be carried out.

Christine also has some circulatory problems as evident from the low blood pressure. The release of histamine that occurs during anaphylaxis has potent vasodilatory effects and therefore has the potential to cause a significant drop in blood pressure. Insertion of a wide-bore IV cannula should therefore be considered and fluid resuscitation administered (Linton and Watson 2010). According to the Resuscitation Council (UK) (2008), it is important to give a rapid IV fluid challenge of 500–1000 mL in an adult in the first instance and administer further doses if required based on the response. It has also been identified that there is no evidence to support the use of colloids over crystalloid infusions (Resuscitation Council (UK) 2008).

4 **Explain the effects of adrenaline in treating anaphylaxis.**

A Adrenaline is the recommended first-line treatment for anaphylaxis. According to the Resuscitation Council (UK) (2008), there are no randomized controlled trials to support its use; however, there is consistent anecdotal evidence that indicate its value in alleviating breathing difficulties and restoring cardiac output. Adrenaline has both alpha and beta effects. Stimulation of alpha adrenoreceptors increases peripheral vascular resistance, thus improving blood pressure and coronary perfusion, reverses peripheral vasodilation, and reduces angio-oedema. Its beta-receptor effects cause bronchodilation, increase the force of myocardial contraction and reduce the release of inflammatory mediators (McLean-Tooke et al. 2003; Resuscitation Council (UK) 2008). As noted earlier, adrenaline seems to work best when given as early as possible after the onset of the reaction and therefore should be readily available in any clinical area where an anaphylactic reaction could potentially occur (Resuscitation Council (UK) 2008).

> Within minutes of the administration of adrenaline, Christine's symptoms very quickly improved. The swelling around her face subsided and her breathing improved. Her blood pressure also quickly returned to within normal limits.

5 **What other medications may now be considered following this acute emergency episode?**

A Adrenaline is the most important drug for the treatment of an anaphylactic reaction (Resuscitation Council (UK) 2008). Other drugs, however, such as antihistamines and corticosteroids may then be considered as second-line treatment drugs of anaphylaxis. Although these drugs have no actual proven impact on the immediate and dangerous effects of anaphylaxis, they may have some value particularly in alleviating mild allergic reactions of the skin and further reducing anaphylactic symptoms (Brown et al. 2006; Resuscitation Council (UK) 2008). An antihistamine such as chlorphenamine is often prescribed after the initial resuscitation period as it may help to further counter the histamine-mediated vasodilation and bronchoconstriction that occur in anaphylaxis. The dose given depends on age. As Christine is 17 years old, the recommended dose for her would therefore be 10 mg and the drug can be given IM or slowly IV. A corticosteroid such as hydrocortisone is also recommended after the resuscitation period as it is thought that it may prevent or shorten protracted reactions. In particular, corticosteroid therapy is believed to perhaps be of particular benefit to patients such as Christine who have a history of asthma (Resuscitation Council (UK) 2008). The dose of hydrocortisone that should be prescribed is also age-dependent and, therefore, in the case of Christine, 200 mg IM or slowly IV would be the recommended amount. Other key drugs that may be considered include bronchodilators such as salbutamol (inhaled or IV) or ipratropium bromide (inhaled). Again, because Christine has a history of asthma, bronchodilator therapy may prove to be particularly beneficial (Bryant 2007; Resuscitation Council (UK) 2008).

6 **What follow-up care should be given to Christine once she has recovered from this event?**

A
- *Routine investigations*: As with all patients who have experienced a medical emergency, appropriate routine investigations will need to be carried out such as a 12-lead ECG, chest X-ray, urea and electrolytes, and arterial blood gas analysis.
- *Mast cell tryptase*: In anaphylaxis, mast cell degranulation leads to markedly increased blood tryptase levels, and therefore obtaining tryptase levels is useful in the follow-up period of suspected anaphylactic reactions in order to help confirm the diagnosis. However, it is important to be aware that the timing of obtaining the sample is crucial as tryptase concentrations in the blood may not increase significantly until at least 30 minutes after the onset of symptoms and the concentrations may be back to normal again within 6-8 hours. Therefore as a minimum, it is recommended that one sample is obtained 1–2 hours after symptoms first present. However, ideally it is recommended that it would be better if three-timed samples were taken as these provide better specificity and sensitivity than a single measurement alone in the confirmation of anaphylaxis (Jevon 2010). The following serial sample procedure is therefore recommended:
  - initial sample: to be taken as soon as possible after resuscitation has started but ensuring that resuscitation is not delayed to take the sample;
  - second sample: 1–2 hours after the start of symptoms;
  - third sample: 24 hours later in order to obtain a baseline tryptase level (Resuscitation Council (UK) 2008).
- *Follow-up observation*: Although most anaphylactic reactions respond rapidly to treatment and do not recur (uniphasic reactions), an observation period is still recommended following the event. This is because symptoms may fail to improve or may worsen once the effects of adrenaline wear off (known as protracted anaphylaxis) or indeed may return after early resolution (biphasic reaction) (Brown et al. 2006). In view of this, patients should be observed for a minimum of 6 hours in a clinical area with facilities for treating life-threatening ABC problems. In some cases, this may even be extended for up to 24 hours, for example, if a reaction occurred in a patient with severe asthma or if a patient had a previous history of biphasic reactions. In this case, Christine appeared to respond well to the treatment for anaphylaxis. However, given that she already has airway and breathing problems due to the quinsy infection, she will require further close monitoring until the acute infection subsides.
- *Pre-discharge education*: All patients who have had an anaphylactic reaction should be reviewed by a senior clinician and given clear instructions to return to hospital if symptoms return (Resuscitation Council (UK) 2008). However, as already noted, given Christine's quinsy infection, she will be required to remain in hospital in any case until the infection clears up. Nevertheless, prior to discharge, Christine should still receive education on the symptoms associated with anaphylaxis and the importance of seeking help early if such a scenario were to arise again.
- *Consider an adrenaline auto-injector*: An auto-injector is often considered for patients at increased risk of an idiopathic anaphylactic reaction or at continued high risk of reactions, such as those whose triggers are venom stings or induced by certain foods. An auto-injector is therefore not usually given to patients such as Christine who have suffered a drug-induced anaphylaxis unless it is thought that it would be difficult to avoid the drug (Resuscitation Council (UK) 2008). Ideally all patients should therefore be assessed by an

allergy specialist and have a treatment plan outlined based on their individual case in order to prevent further episodes from occurring (Jevon 2010).

Key points

- Anaphylaxis is a life-threatening medical emergency.
- Prompt assessment and management using the ABCDE approach are important in order to diagnose and manage anaphylaxis appropriately.
- In particular, early access to help and prompt administration of adrenaline are vital.

REFERENCES

Brown, S.G.A., Mullins, R.J. and Gold, M.S. (2006) Anaphylaxis: diagnosis and management, *The Medical Journal of Australia*, 185(5): 283–9.

Bryant, H. (2007) Anaphylaxis: recognition, treatment and education, *Emergency Nurse*, 15(2): 24–8.

East, L. (2010) Acute emergency situations, in F. Creed and C. Spiers (eds) *Care of the Acutely Ill Adult*. Oxford: Oxford University Press.

Jevon, P. (2010) Recognition and treatment of anaphylaxis in hospital, *British Journal of Nursing*, 19(16): 1015–20.

Linton, E. and Watson, D. (2010) Recognition, assessment and management of anaphylaxis, *Nursing Standard*, 24(46): 35–9.

McLean-Tooke, A.P.C., Bethune, C.A., Fay, A.C. and Spickett, G.P. (2003) Adrenaline in the treatment of anaphylaxis: what is the evidence? *British Medical Journal*, 327(7427): 1332–5.

Resuscitation Council (UK) (2008) *Emergency Treatment of Anaphylactic Reactions. Guidelines for Healthcare Providers*. London: Resuscitation Council (UK).

Royal College of Physicians (2009) *New Guidance to Address Soaring Numbers of Allergic Reactions*. Available at: http://bit.ly/9s9QfP (accessed 12 December 2011).

CASE STUDY 17
Burns
Niall McKenna

Case outline

Patrick Jones, a 56-year-old gentleman, has been admitted to A&E having been rescued from a house fire. He arrives into the resuscitation area having been treated by the paramedic crew at the scene. He is drowsy but rousable on admission and has high flow oxygen via a non-rebreath mask in situ, intravenous (IV) access has been established and IV fluids are in progress. He appears quite dyspnoeic on arrival.

---

1 **Outline the action required to comprehensively assess and manage Patrick's current health status on arrival at A&E. Provide a rationale for your responses.**

A Table 17.1 shows the ABCDE procedure to follow when dealing with burns.

Table 17.1 The ABCDE procedure in the case of burns

Assessment	Initial management strategies
Immediate Airway/Breathing/ Circulation assessment is of major consideration for all severe burns (Greaves et al. 2009)	Significant airway obstruction as a result of upper/ lower respiratory tract burn injury will compromise airway patency, leading to hypoxia and potential cardiorespiratory arrest
Obtain history and confirm the interventions undertaken in the pre-hospital setting	Establishing pertinent history and clinical presentation will assist clinicians in the triage process and guide immediate treatment. Detailed history may identify possible blast injury or possible exposure to other types of burn injury including those of a chemical or electrical nature
A = Airway	**Airway Management**
Signs of airway compromise in the initial assessment necessitate continuous airway evaluation and definitive management. Ensuring immediate patency of the airway is essential given the potential for development of upper airway oedema	All patients with serious burn injury should have high flow oxygen 85% at 15 L administered via humidified non-rebreath mask to maintain oxygen saturations >96% or 100% oxygen if an endotracheal tube is in situ. Humidification of oxygen therapy will prevent drying and sloughing of the mucosa (Hettiaratchy and Papini 2004a)

(Continued overleaf)

Table 17.1 (*Continued*)

Assessment	Initial management strategies
Assess patient's ability to communicate Assess for signs of angio-oedema (swollen tongue/lips), obstruction (blood/secretions/broken teeth/tissue injury) secondary to upper airway/facial trauma	Presence of abnormal breathing sounds, wheeze, stridor or gurgling noises, cyanotic lips/tongue, difficulties in communication (incomplete/short sentences) may indicate a compromised airway (Resuscitation Council (UK) 2011)
Observe for carbonaceous sputum, singed nasal/facial hairs and blistering around upper airway. Observe for a change in voice/hoarseness or harsh cough	Maintain airway patency utilizing appropriate airway adjuncts if required Excessive airway secretions should be removed to facilitate reduced respiratory congestion and ensure patency of airway adjuncts
Inhalation of hot gases in the form of flame or smoke may cause injury to the upper airway resulting in oedema that may develop over a period of hours following inhalation causing airway occlusion (Kasten et al. 2011)	Preparation for endotracheal intubation or tracheostomy formation will be required in the event of a compromised airway and reduced respiratory functioning (Hettiaratchy and Papini 2004a) If airway oedema precludes intubation a surgical airway may be required (tracheostomy, cricothyroidotomy) (Greaves et al. 2009)
B = Breathing	**Respiratory management**
Evidence of duskiness/cyanosis in lips/tongue/ear lobes Respiratory rate/depth/pattern Assess mechanics of breathing, i.e. bilateral/symmetrical chest wall rising Assess accessory muscle use	Assessment and continuous monitoring of respiratory status is important to facilitate evaluation of overall respiratory function and response to treatment
Tracheal deviation Seesaw pattern	Paradoxical/abnormal breathing mechanics or tracheal deviation may indicate the presence of tension pneumothorax, haemothorax or flail chest which may be secondary to blast injury from exploding volatile materials. This may require the insertion or a chest drain.
Mechanical restriction of breathing	Deep dermal or full thickness circumferential burns of the chest can limit chest excursion and prevent adequate ventilation This may require escharotomies in severe cases
Chest X-ray/computed tomography (CT)	Chest X-ray or CT – to evaluate/confirm the impact of trauma to thorax

Pulse oximetry –SpO$_2$
Caution is required in the use of pulse oximetry readings as the presence of carboxyhaemoglobin can undermine the reliability of oximetry readings in highlighting oxygen saturations (Hettiaratchy and Papini 2004a)

Given the affinity of carbon monoxide (CO) to displace oxygen from the haemoglobin molecule and its slow disassociation (half-life 4 hours), patients with suspected exposure to CO should receive high flow oxygen via a non-rebreath mask initially as indicated above

Arterial blood gases

Use of arterial blood gases (ABGs) when patient is critical can assess respiratory function, gaseous exchange PaO$_2$, PaCO$_2$, given the potential inhalation of noxious gases

Auscultation

Identifies air entry/presence of crackles/breath sounds to recognize alterations in upper/lower airway

Percussion

Examination of thoracic resonance in the absence of radiological testing can highlight the presence of respiratory complications (Resuscitation Council United Kingdom (UK) 2011; American College of Surgeons 2008)

C = Circulation

Circulatory management

Pulse rate (peripheral/central), rhythm and amplitude
Check pulse in affected limbs
Check peripheral circulation for signs of deficit. Any peripheral circumferential burn can act as a tourniquet especially once oedema develops after fluid resuscitation

Haemodynamic assessment following burn injury is essential given the potential for haemodynamic compromise due to fluid loss. Continuous monitoring of cardiovascular observations will highlight potential deterioration in circulatory status, identify potential arrhythmias and evaluate the efficacy of interventions

Evaluate affected limbs to assess circulation/blood flow – compare with corresponding limb
Capillary refill time (CRT) (central)
Blood pressure

Circulatory assessment may also identify physiological compensatory mechanisms in the presence of injury including BP and pulse responses or delayed capillary refill time

IV access to peripheral veins

Secure intravenous (IV) access with a wide-bore cannula preferably placed through unburnt tissue is required to facilitate rapid fluid resuscitation

Baseline bloods, full blood picture (FBP), urea and electrolytes, clotting screen. Blood group and hold or cross-match serum (Hettiaratchy and Papini 2004a)

Reservation of key bloods will provide a baseline to guide fluid replacement therapy and identify multi-systemic effects of burn injury. FBP is significant to identify haemoglobin/platelets and white cell count indicating cellular losses and the potential development of infection due to high risk of microbial infection

(Continued overleaf)

Table 17.1 (*Continued*)

Assessment	Initial management strategies
	Identification of blood group and rhesus status will ensure safe and effective delivery of blood products if required in fluid management/resuscitation
Obtain ECG Place patient on a cardiac monitor	To rule out cardiac arrhythmias induced by fluid and electrolyte loss and potential effects of electrical injury
Urinary catheterization	Measuring urinary output (0.5 mL/kg/hour in adults) will indicate renal function/perfusion in the presence of hypovolaemia and monitor the effects of fluid resuscitation
Central venous pressure monitoring	CVP monitoring allows for an accurate assessment of haemodynamics if hypovolaemic shock is present and large volumes of fluid are required for resuscitation

D = Disability

AVPU (*Alert, responsive to Voice, Pain or Unresponsive*)	Continuing neurological assessment is important to identify potential neurological deficit resulting from inhalation injury and levels of carboxyhaemoglobin
Glasgow Coma Scale (GCS) Pupillary check – size, equality and reaction to light	AVPU will indicate gross neurological damage only and is appropriate in the primary survey. Glasgow Coma Scale may wait until secondary assessment
Blood glucose measurement Alterations in blood glucose levels may begin to rise initially as metabolic changes, secondary to systemic injury takes hold (Kasten et al. 2011)	Maintain blood sugar within normal limits with the use of insulin therapy if required
Check for medication history if possible	A knowledge of present medication history will assist in the ongoing management of the patient
Pain assessment Pain assessment utilizing a recognized pain scoring tool may indicate extent of burn injury and the presence of concomitant injuries endured as a result of involvement in the fire including trauma (American College of Surgeons 2008)	*Pain management* Superficial burns can be extremely painful. All patients with severe burns should receive intravenous morphine at a dose appropriate to body weight unless contraindicated. Regular reassessment is necessary to evaluate the effectiveness of treatment. Consideration must be given to the fact that the severely burned patient may be restless secondary to hypoxia rather than pain – caution must be exercised with respect to the potential for analgesics or sedation to mask the signs of neurological or circulatory deterioration (Hettiaratchy and Papini 2004a)

E = Exposure

Head-to-toe examination of patient for assessment of burn depth and extent (total body surface area, TBSA) utilizing an objective assessment tool

Assessment of extent of burn depth and severity will guide initial management of the patient. It is important to check for concomitant injuries during this examination. During the assessment the environment should be kept warm, with small areas of skin exposed sequentially to minimize heat loss and maximize patient dignity (Morton et al. 2005). Hypothermia will lead to hypoperfusion and deepening of burn wounds

---

2   **Consider the assessment of the depth and extent of the burn injury that Patrick has sustained in the fire.**

A   Injury to the integument will be dependent on the level of exposure and type of burn injury sustained, i.e. thermal, chemical or electrical. Damage to the skin often can be classified into differing zones of damage as described by Jackson in 1947 including:

- *Zone of coagulation*: This is the zone of maximum tissue damage. The damage is irreversible with coagulation of constituent proteins (thermal/electrical burns).
- *Zone of stasis*: This zone is identified with decreased tissue perfusion but is potentially salvageable if fluid resuscitation is successful.
- *Zone of hyperaemia*: Tissue perfusion is increased in this zone following the burn injury and the area will usually recover unless severe sepsis or hypoperfusion develops (McCance and Huether, 2010).

Assessment of the total body surface area (TBSA) involved in the burn is important to assist in calculating fluid resuscitation therapy. In addition, the type and location of the injury as well as the patient's age and medical history are also significant considerations (Urden et al. 2006).

EXTENT OF BURN INJURY

There are three commonly used methods of estimating the extent of burn surface areas; however, each of the methods has advantages and disadvantages.

1   *Rule of palms* (palmar surface): A patient's palm is considered to be approximately 0.8%– 1% of TBSA. This can be used to estimate the area of relatively small burns or very large burns if the amount of unburnt skin is assessed (Kirby and Blackburn 1987). It is inaccurate for medium-sized burn areas (Williams 2009). However, in appropriate circumstances, usually pre-admission or in a triage setting, it is a quick and relatively easy method of assessment.

2   *Wallace rule of nines*: This is a simple and common formula which divides areas of the body into 9% and 18% respectively. Each arm is 9% body surface area (BSA), each leg is 18%, anterior trunk 18%, posterior trunk 18%, head 9% and perineum 1% It is useful in estimating the size of medium to large burns in adults (Kyle and Wallace 1951).

3   *Lund and Browder chart*: In the hospital setting this is the most accurate and accepted method of assessing the area involved in the burn as it compensates for variation in body shape with age (Lund and Browder 1944). It will provide an accurate assessment of burns area in children. However, it is time-consuming and requires some expertise to complete so it is often reserved for use once a patient is admitted to a specialist burns unit.

DEPTH OF BURN INJURY

In current practice, burn injuries are classified as superficial, partial thickness or full thickness. Accurate assessment of burn depth on admission is important in making decisions about future wound care and management (Papini 2004).

Superficial burns

Superficial burns by definition affect only the epidermal layer of the skin and are typified by the presence of erythema. Blistering may occur but is not common. Supportive therapy is usually all that is required to address the pain which can be experienced by the patient. Healing occurs rapidly by regeneration from undamaged keratinocytes within the basal layers of the skin.

Partial thickness burns

*   *Superficial partial thickness* burns affecting the dermis and epidermis are often characterized by blistering and more intense levels of pain as nerve endings may be exposed. Healing can take place within two weeks, facilitated by the regeneration of keratinocytes from sebaceous and follicular tissue. Treatment is aimed at preventing wound progression by maintaining a warm moist healing environment.
*   *Deep partial thickness* injury extends further into dermal tissue affecting greater levels of subcutaneous structures including sebaceous glands and hair follicles. Initially skin appears red with patchy white areas although the appearance may change over time. Given the deeper injury, healing is slower and may be characterized by scarring and contraction of tissues leading to loss of function (Urden et al. 2006).

Full thickness burns

These burns involve all layers of dermal tissue and associated structures including blood vessels, lymphatic supply and nerve endings. Healing only occurs from the edges of the wound and therefore will be prolonged in the absence of debridement and will require skin grafting. Considerable contraction may be evident, particularly over joints. The wound may have a black, cherry-red or perhaps dry/leathery appearance. There may be associated loss of thermoregulatory function and potential hypothermia with no pain sensation evident (Evers et al. 2010).

Most patients presenting with burn injury will have mixed areas of different burn depth within the overall surface area affected. Establishing burn depth will consider a number of approaches including the needle prick test – brisk bleeding is indicative of superficial injury, delayed bleeding suggests a deep dermal burn, with no bleeding evident in full thickness injury. Sensation and pain will indicate superficial to partial thickness burns with the absence of pain indicating full thickness injury. Appearance of the burn injury may contribute to establishing extent of burn injury (Hettiaratchy and Papini 2004b). It should be noted, however, that assessment of burn depth is challenging even for experienced clinical staff.

Following the initial assessment it is established that Patrick has suffered a range of burns, both deep dermal and full thickness to approximately 25% of his body surface area. His lower arms are reddened and swollen with some injuries on his hands appearing cherry red *and* leathery. Extensive blistering is noted around the remaining skin on the hands and arms.

Vital signs:
Airway: lips swollen, stridor and discoloured sputum noted.
Respiratory rate: 29 breaths per minute, regular, symmetrical movements of lung fields
   but evident use of accessory muscles.
SpO_2: 83% (on high concentration oxygen), 78 % (in room air)
Heart rate: 120 beats per minute (irregular)
Blood pressure: 97/50 mmHg
Temperature: 35.5°C
AVPU: 'V'
Glasgow Coma Scale: 14/15
Blood glucose: 10 mmol/L (no history of diabetes mellitus)
Pain score: 10/10

---

3   **Given Patrick's clinical presentation, explain how burn injury may lead to systemic alterations in body functioning from a physiological perspective. What clinical signs might be identified in the acute phase of his injury?**

A   # CLINICAL SIGNS

Susceptibility to infection

The presence of a significant burn will have an impact on the body's non-specific and specific defences. As one essential function of the skin is to protect underlying tissues from trauma, loss of bodily fluids and infection, the absence of the physical barrier permits an extensive site of entry for invading pathogens.

Burn injury will diminish the population of both fixed and free macrophages which will limit the body's ability to remove necrotic tissue and pathogens. Loss of neutrophils, eosinophils, and monocytes will impair the body's ability to fight infection. The absence of macrophages will affect the ability of interferons to slow the spread of infection.

Immunologic response to burn injury is immediate, prolonged and severe – immunosuppression with increased susceptibility to potentially fatal systemic burn wound sepsis may develop (McCance and Huether 2010).

Fluid and electrolyte homeostasis

Burn injury results in dramatic changes in most physiological functions of the body within the first few minutes after the event. The effect of the burn depends on the extent of the body surface area and the depth of the cutaneous injury involved.

The acute physiologic result of a major burn (≥25% TBSA) results in life-threatening hypovolaemic shock. Damaged circulation within the dermis and hypodermic layers results in massive fluid losses from the circulating volume due to increased capillary endothelial permeability as a result of both the burn damage and the consequent inflammatory process. This will be evidenced by the development of hypotension coupled with hyperviscosity in the remaining vascular circulation. Alterations in full blood count will be evident as cells are lost through the damaged capillaries.

In the initial stages of burn shock, there is a shift of electrolytes including potassium, sodium, calcium, chloride, magnesium, phosphate and a fluid shift of H_2O and albumin from the capillary into the extra-vascular space and the external environment, leading to a decrease in colloid osmotic pressure and widespread oedema. Intra-cellular H_2O and Na increase during the acute hypovolaemic period.

Loss of electrolyte homeostasis results in impaired cellular metabolism, cell membrane permeability is altered and results in prolongation of depolarization and repolarization times as the sodium–potassium pump is impaired. This will impact primarily on cardiac muscle and skeletal muscle functioning, leading to potential arrhythmias and cardiac dysfunction. This may be reflected in ECG abnormalities and decreased neurological functioning which will ultimately affect the patient's level of consciousness

Renal function

Stimulation of compensatory mechanisms to maintain homeostasis occurs following the burn injury including the renin–angiotensin system to try and compensate for renal hypoperfusion. This leads to decreased urinary output <30 mL/hr and deranged electrolyte balance in an effort to conserve fluid.

Acute renal failure may develop if hypoperfusion of the kidney is sustained affecting glomerular filtration rate. In addition, hyperviscosity of blood and destruction of red blood cells results in acute tubular necrosis.

Cardiovascular system

Capillary permeability is increased by the release of cytokines and other inflammatory mediators, leading to loss of intravascular proteins and fluids into the interstitial compartment with evidence of massive oedema formation and hypovolaemia.

Myocardial contractility is decreased, possibly due to the release of tumour necrosis factor-alpha and reactive oxygen radicals (myocardial depressant factor).

These changes, coupled with fluid loss from the burn wound, result in systemic hypotension and end organ hypoperfusion. Compensatory mechanisms are initiated in attempt to correct fluid shifts/loss and include tachycardia and reduced capillary refill times.

Peripheral and splanchnic vasoconstriction occurs to redirect blood supply to vital organs leading to a reduction in peristalsis with loss of gut motility. This may result in translocation of bacteria across the gut wall causing sepsis (Hettiaratchy and Dziewulski 2004).

Respiratory system

There are several ways in which burn injury can compromise respiration.

- *Mechanical restriction*: Deep dermal or full thickness circumferential burns of the chest can limit chest excursion and prevent adequate ventilation. Angio-oedema may occur secondary to the inflammatory response. Clinical features associated with compromise in the respiratory system include tachypnoea/bradypnoea, dyspnoea, stridor/wheeze, cyanosis. Deranged ABGs will reveal acidosis. Possible blast injury can compromise ventilation with the potential development of tension pneumothoraces, contusions and alveolar trauma and can lead to adult respiratory distress syndrome and possible respiratory arrest (Hettiaratchy and Dziewulski 2004).
- *Smoke inhalation*: The products of combustion, e.g. chemicals and soot, when cooled act as direct irritants, leading to bronchospasm, inflammation and excessive pulmonary oedema, resulting in excess production of secretions and hypoxia. The presence of carbonaceous sputum and a change in voice/cough are indicative of smoke inhalation. Inhalation injury may have damaged the mucociliary escalator which may exacerbate the situation as pulmonary secretions are retained – atelectasis or pneumonia may follow.
- *Carboxyhaemoglobin*: Carbon monoxide binds to deoxyhaemoglobin with 40 times the affinity of oxygen. It also binds with the cytochrome oxidase pathway (intercellular proteins). These two effects lead to intercellular and extracellular hypoxia (Hettiaratchy and Papini 2004). Increased carboxyhaemoglobin levels will result in drowsiness/confusion/agitation.

Metabolic activity

The basal metabolic rate (BMR) increases up to three times its original baseline rate due to alterations in sympathetic nervous activity and an increase and resetting of the body's thermal regulatory point to facilitate extensive wound repair. Tachycardia, tachypnoea and hyperpyrexia are associated with this increase in BMR.

Catecholamines are released in large quantities – cortisol, glucagon and insulin levels are elevated in response to this, which increases gluconeogenesis, lipolysis and proteolysis resulting in hyperglycaemia. The process of hypermetabolism is augmented by high levels of cytokines, oxygen radicals and chemotactic factors.

Catabolism will ensue without intervention leading to latent cachexia/muscle wasting (Evers et al. 2010).

4 **Given the extent of the burn injury revealed in Patrick's initial assessment, outline the key priorities and interventions in his ongoing acute management.**

A Table 17.2 shows the priorities and interventions required.

Table 17.2 Priority and interventions in burns cases

Priority	Interventions	Rationale
Urgent fluid resuscitation	Commencement of IV fluids (crystalloids, e.g. Hartmann's solution) as per fluid resuscitation formula, e.g. Baxter (Parkland) formula (Adult) Total fluid requirement in 24 hours: 4 mL × percentage of total burn surface area × body weight (kg) 50% of volume administered in first 8 hours. It is worth noting that the time dependent variable for all formulae begins from the time of injury (Williams 2009) Remaining 50% in next 16 hours (Morton et al. 2005) Any resuscitation formula provides only an estimate of fluid need and local policy should be consulted in regard to recommended formulae and fluids to be used Monitor effects of fluid resuscitation by observing urinary output Expected urinary output of 0.5–1.0 mL/kg/hour in adults	Potential fluid losses must be replaced so that homoeostasis is maintained, thus reducing the risk of multi-organ failure secondary to hypovolaemia. There is a range of potential fluid resuscitation regimes and their efficacy must be measured in response to physiological stabilization from time of injury. While crystalloids are recommended in initial fluid resuscitation, consideration may be given to other fluid types to facilitate glucose and protein maintenance or levels of packed cell volume. Colloid infusion maybe commenced following the first 24 hours. Monitoring urinary output is essential in assessing effectiveness of fluid resuscitation and renal perfusion given the potential for hypovolaemic shock (Greaves et al. 2009)
Pain management	Cover all exposed burned areas with non-adhesive coverings following initial assessment	Covering affected areas of burned skin will deflect air currents passing over exposed nerve endings especially in partial thickness burns thus reducing levels of pain experienced

	Continue to evaluate the efficacy of the pain management strategy utilizing a pain tool	Superficial and partial thickness burns are often extremely painful, thus patients with large burns should continue to receive titrated dosages of IV opioid analgesia appropriate to body weight to manage ongoing pain intensity
Wound management	Undertake comprehensive wound assessment establishing depth, extent, location and nature of burn injury utilizing an objective assessment tool (Wallace rule of nines, Rule of palms or Lund and Browder)	Effective wound management has a beneficial effect on overall outcome and subsequent scarring thus contributing to the reduction of psychosocial effects related to burn injury (Rowley-Conwy 2010)
	Cooling of burn injury (avoiding excessive cooling) as per local protocol (Water-Jel or sterile saline)	Cooling burn injury will limit the extent of tissue damage and aid initial pain relief. Application of cold water or compresses in patients with extensive burns, however, may induce hypothermia and prolong ischaemia in zones of hyperaemia at sites of injury
	Cover affected areas with non-adhesive gauze as per local policy (e.g. Jelonet). Consideration must be given to the application of occlusive and/or secondary dressings if high levels of exudate are present	Covering affected areas with non-adhesive gauze will protect areas subject to trauma and will facilitate early inspection without changing the appearance of the wound. The use of occlusive dressings also inhibits evaporative losses, minimizes pain and establishes a moist environment to promote healing
	Referral to burns centre	Input from specialist burns centres will facilitate accurate assessment and management of complex burn injury, instigating specialist intervention
	Observe for early complications/ signs of infection Provide tetanus prophylaxis (Kasten et al. 2011)	Damage to integument's protective function may lead to development of wound infection and sepsis. Given the extensive nature of this patient's burn injury (20% TBSA), the development of systemic complications is a major risk

REFERENCES

American College of Surgeons Committee on Trauma (2008) *Advanced Trauma Life Support for Doctors*, 8th edn. Washington, DC: American College of Surgeons.

Evers, L.H., Bhavsar, D. and Mailander, P. (2010) The biology of burn injury, *Experimental Dermatology*, 19: 777–83.

Greaves, I., Porter, K. and Ryan, J. (eds) (2009) *Trauma Care Manual,* 2nd edn. New York: Arnold.

Hettiaratchy, S. and Dziewulski, P. (2004) ABC of burns: pathophysiology and types of burns, *British Medical Journal*, 328: 1427–9.

Hettiaratchy, S. and Papini, R. (2004a) ABC of burns: initial management of a major burn: I – overview, *British Medical Journal*, 328: 1555–7.

Hettiaratchy, S. and Papini, R. (2004b) ABC of burns: initial management of a major burn: II – assessment and resuscitation, *British Medical Journal*, 329: 101–3.

Kasten, K.R., Makley, A.T. and Kagan, R.J. (2011) Update on the critical care management of severe burns, *Journal of Intensive Care Medicine*, 26(4): 223–6.

Kirby, N.G. and Blackburn, G. (eds) (1987) *Field Surgery Pocket Book*. London: HMSO.

Kyle, M.J. and Wallace, A.B. (1951) Fluid replacement in burnt children, *British Journal of Plastic Surgery*, 3:194–204.

Lund, C.C. and Browder, N.C. (1944) Estimation of area of burns, *Surgery, Gynaecology and Obstetrics*, 79: 352–8.

McCance, K.L. and Huether, S.E. (2010) *Pathophysiology: The Biological Basis for Disease in Adults and Children*, 6th edn. St Louis, MO: Mosby Elsevier.

Morton, P.G., Fontaine, D.K., Hudak, C.M. and Gallo, B.M. (eds) (2005) *Critical Care Nursing: A Holistic Approach*, 8th edn. Philadelphia, PA: Lippincott Williams and Wilkins.

Papini, R. (2004) ABC of burns: management of burn injuries of various depth, *British Medical Journal*, 329: 158–60.

Resuscitation Council (UK) (2011) *Advanced Life Support*, 6th edn. London: Resuscitation Council.

Rowley-Conwy, G. (2010) Infection prevention and treatment in patients with major burn injuries, *Nursing Standard*, 25(7) 51–60.

Urden L.D., Stacy, K.M. and Lough, M.E. (2006) *Critical Care Nursing: Diagnosis and Management*, 5th edn. St Louis, MO: Mosby Elsevier.

Williams, C. (2009) Successful assessment and management of burn injuries, *Nursing Standard*, 23(32): 53–62.

Index

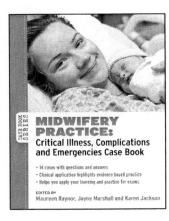

MIDWIFERY PRACTICE
Critical Illness, Complications and Emergencies Case Book

Maureen Raynor, Jayne Marshall and Karen Jackson

9780335242733 (Paperback)
May 2012

eBook also available

Part of a case book series, this book contains 14 common pregnancy and childbirth emergency scenarios to help prepare student midwives for life in practice. Each case explores and explains the pathology, pharmacology and care principles, and uses test questions and answers to help assess learning.

Key features:

- Covers the principles, pathology and skills involved in a range of birthing scenarios
- Each chapter includes Q&A's, further resources, pre-requisite learning, summaries, boxes and learning tools in order to track and further learning
- The practical cases will help you link theory to practice

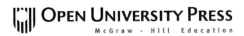

OPEN UNIVERSITY PRESS
McGraw - Hill Education

www.openup.co.uk

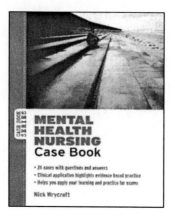

MENTAL HEALTH NURSING CASE BOOK

Nick Wrycraft

9780335242955 (Paperback)
September 2012

eBook also available

This case book is aimed at mental health nursing students and those going into mental health settings, such as social workers. The cases include a wide range of mental health diagnoses from common problems such as anxiety or depression through to severe and enduring conditions such as schizophrenia. The cases will be organised into sections by life stage from childhood through to old age.

Key features:

- Uses a case study approach which provides a realistic context that students will find familiar
- Each case study will commence with a practice focused scenario
- Provides a commentary offering insights, perspectives and references to theories, research and further explanations and discussion

www.openup.co.uk

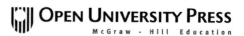

OPEN UNIVERSITY PRESS

McGraw - Hill Education